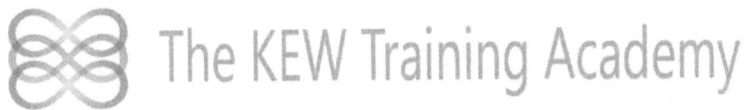

Hypnotherapy Practitioner Course

Professional Accredited Hypnotherapy Training

The KEW Training Academy

8 Stockley Mews

Shevington

Wigan

WN6 8AN

Telephone: 0161 408 2814

www.kewtrainingacademy.com

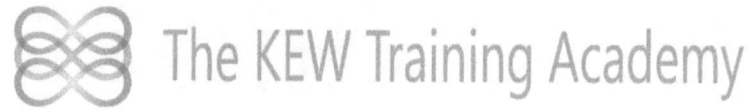

The KEW Training Academy

The KEW Training Academy was established in 2006 by Karen E Wells to fill a gap in the market for Hypnotherapy Training Courses, both Classroom based and Online that combined Hypnosis with Regression & Healing.

Having successfully helped hundreds of clients over the years and trained other therapists in these areas of expertise around the world, The KEW Training Academy offers easy and effective solutions that work for your client either personally or professionally.

Your course has been tailored from years of experience enabling you to achieve the goals that give you and your client's the key to freedom.

The Key to Freedom, is Unlocking The Subconscious Mind

Karen E Wells

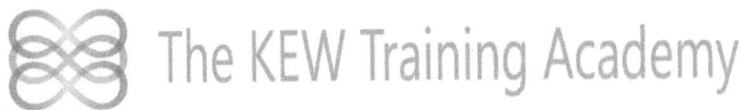

Welcome – Hypnotherapy Practitioners Course

Welcome to your Hypnotherapy Practitioners Course. This course includes your full Hypnotherapy Practitioner Training Manual, Hypnosis Scripts, Inductions & Consultation Forms.

At the end of this course you will find the course assessment paper, which you should complete and send back to me via the post or email. This will then be assessed and upon successful completion, you will receive your Hypnotherapy certificate. This course contains everything you need to get you from the sofa to being the therapist in your area.

Included as an additional bonus is a Ultimate Relaxation MP3 – which comes as part of this package – this will give you an idea of how to construct a Hypnotherapy session; The Induction, The Deepener The Therapeutic Session and bringing your client back to full conscious awareness. In 8 minutes, your client can be in a world of relaxed bliss!

Please join our Facebook page for regular updates & support:
https://www.facebook.com/pages/The-KEW-Training-Academy/189715934386898

Welcome to the world of Hypnotherapy.

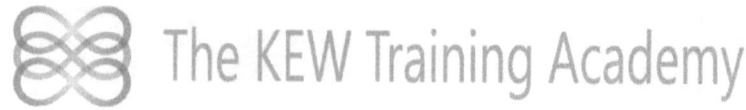
The KEW Training Academy

Contents:

Hypnotherapy Practitioner Course - Professional Accredited Hypnotherapy Training

Hypnotherapy Practitioner Course - Professional Accredited Hypnotherapy Training

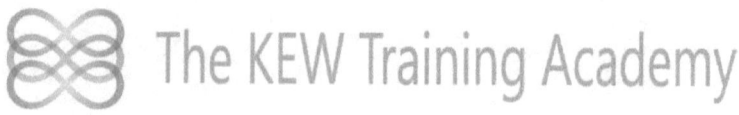
The KEW Training Academy

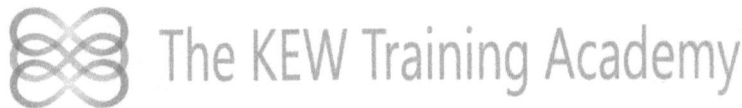

Introducing Hypnosis

Hypnosis is often associated with stage shows and other often mystical things. Hypnosis is not at all mystical and is a perfectly natural state of mind that we all go into hundreds of times every day.

Have you ever experienced driving in your car but not knowing the exact things you did (like every turn of the indicator or wheel for example) – this is because you would have been in a very light hypnotic state. On a sub conscious level, you were still in control of the vehicle you were driving. The same happens when you are focussed intensely on a movie or book, just that slight shift of awareness from your normal conscious state and that is Hypnosis.

Hypnosis

The term Hypnosis comes from the Greek word "Hypnos" meaning sleep. Here are a few of the many definitions of Hypnosis:

- Focussed consciousness
- An altered state of consciousness
- Extreme relaxation
- Guided Meditation
- A series of instructions

"In therapy, Hypnosis usually involves the person experiencing a sense of deep relaxation with their attention focussed inward and appropriate suggestions made by the therapist."

These suggestions help people make positive changes within themselves. In a Hypnotherapy session you are always in control and are not made to do anything. All Hypnosis is Self Hypnosis and a Hypnotherapist just facilitates the client's experience.

Hypnosis Facts

- Hypnosis was accepted by the American Medical Association is 1958.
- Hypnosis is a very natural state of mind and is safe
- No-one has ever been hurt by Hypnosis
- Hypnosis is not mind control

Hypnotherapy Practitioner Course - Professional Accredited Hypnotherapy Training

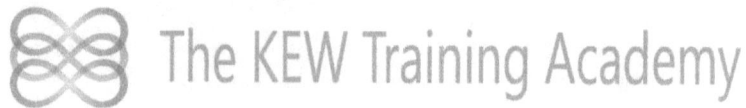

- You cannot get stuck in Hypnosis – this has never happened to anyone

- The worst case scenario is that you fall asleep

- Hypnosis is focused consciousness

- Sleep is a state of unconsciousness

- The wording of "Sleep" in Hypnosis means close your eyes and go deeply relaxed as if you are asleep

Hypnosis is simply a series of instructions; all you have to do is focus on what the hypnotherapist is saying and follow his or her instructions.

Uses for Hypnosis

Hypnosis is a powerful tool for implementing change within a person's life. Many practitioners frown upon the use of hypnosis in stage shows when the techniques are used in a less serious light.

Stage Hypnosis works where the viewer witness's individuals indulging their sense of humour by believing that he/she has x-ray vision and can see all person's underwear or he/she believes they are deeply in love with a broom. Although this use of hypnosis creates humour, the viewer usually fails to realise the true "power" of hypnosis; a contestant truly believes they have x-ray vision, a physical impossibility.

Paul Mckenna, one of the recent pioneers of hypnosis, no longer carries out stage shows, but prefers the subject matter to be seen in its more serious form in order to give it the credibility it deserves.

Hypnosis is a very natural state of mind. In fact, you enter into a state of hypnosis many times a day. Let me give you some examples:

- You are driving in your car and you almost miss your turn because you are so focused on a specific thought - that is highway hypnosis.

- When you arrive at your destination and don't even remember how you got there because your mind was somewhere else - that is a state of hypnosis.

- If you are watching TV or reading a really good book and someone is talking to you, but you don't hear a word they say because you are so focused on your show – that is a state of hypnosis!

- If you get a bruise or a cut but don't realize it until later (once again because you were so focused on doing something else at the time) that is a state of hypnosis.

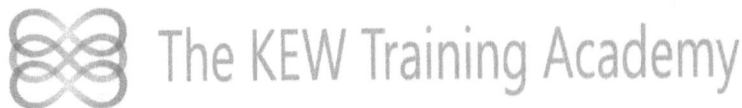
The KEW Training Academy

Definition of Hypnotherapy

Contrary to popular belief, hypnosis is not a state of deep sleep. It does involve the induction of a trance-like condition, but when in it, the patient is actually in an enhanced state of awareness, concentrating entirely on the hypnotist's voice. In this state, the conscious mind is suppressed and the subconscious mind is revealed. The therapist is able to suggest ideas, concepts and lifestyle adaptations to the patient, the seeds of which become firmly planted.

The practice of promoting healing or positive development in any way is known as hypnotherapy. As such, hypnotherapy is a kind of psychotherapy. Hypnotherapy aims to re-program patterns of behaviour within the mind, enabling irrational fears, phobias, negative thoughts and suppressed emotions to be overcome.

As the body is released from conscious control during the relaxed trance-like state of hypnosis, breathing becomes slower and deeper, the pulse rate drops and the metabolic rate falls. Similar changes along nervous pathways and hormonal channels enable the sensation of pain to become less acute, and the awareness of unpleasant symptoms, such as nausea or indigestion, to be alleviated.

How Does It Work?

Hypnosis is thought to work by altering our state of consciousness in such a way that the analytical left-hand side of the brain is turned off, while the non-analytical right-hand side is made more alert.

The conscious control of the mind is inhibited, and the subconscious mind awoken. Since the subconscious mind is a deeper-seated, more instinctive force than the conscious mind, this is the part which has to change for the patient's behaviour and physical state to alter.

For example, a patient who consciously wants to overcome their fear of spiders may try everything they consciously can to do it, but will still fail as long as their subconscious mind retains this terror and prevents the patient from succeeding.

Progress can only be made by reprogramming the subconscious so that deep-seated instincts and beliefs are abolished or altered.

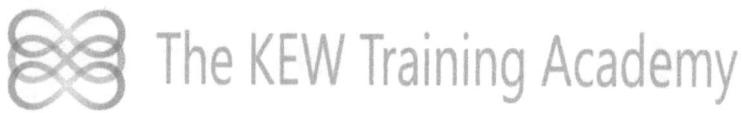

The KEW Training Academy

The 7 Principals of Hypnosis

In Hypnosis, there are 7 methods commonly used. These are important aspects for you to consider whenever you are about to start a Hypnotherapy Session.

- Collaboration: *You Need Their Help Too* – Your client needs to be at a point in their life where they are ready to undertake the changes that may happen resulting from the session you will do with them. A strong conscious mind can overrule your suggestions or the work you are doing. For a successful session, the client must be ready and willing to take their own journey.

- Forced cognition: *Saying It Makes Them Think It* – When you use Suggestion Therapy, you will making suggestions to the subconscious mind, this then makes the client have new thought patterns and to be able to successfully reach their goals.

- Sensory thought: *Thinking About Events Triggers Senses* – Using the skills you will learn from this course, you can take your clients back into memories. When these memories arise – the senses become more alert and astute, making the whole experience more real.

- Physical thought: *Thinking Changes The Body* – As therapist's we are all aware of the connection between the mind and body – when we connect with what is happening in our bodies, amazing healing can happen.

- Feedback: *Check That It Is Working & Works* – Never be afraid to ask your clients in the session and following up with them after the session, how they have responded and how they are feeling afterwards.

- Utilization: *Make Use Of What Happens. Everything Is A Resource* – Use your client's terminology – their words – we will go into that later – there is no better way of connecting and healing your client than to use the terminology that they themselves tell you.

- Confidence: *The Attitude Of The Therapist Is Key* – One of the most important aspects of being a Hypnotherapist. You must believe yourself that this therapy works, trust it even if your client shows doubt and know that your client chose you on a soul level and that you are meant to work together. Know in the work you have done, that many things physically and energetically have been shifted for your client.

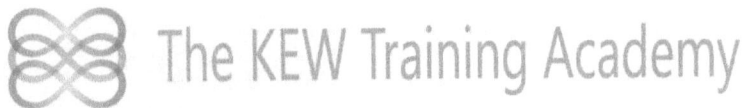

Parts of the Mind

Conscious Mind

There are four parts within the Conscious Mind – *rational, analytical, will power,* and *temporary memory.*

The Conscious Mind is where we spend most of our time, but it is actually the weakest part of our mind. The Conscious Mind is the rational, analytical part of the mind. It's the thinking, judging part of the mind. Humans must have a reason for everything.

Our ability to rationalize our actions is what keeps us sane. For example, a smoker will rationalize his or her actions by saying "smoking helps me relax and focus." The truth is that cigarettes raise heart rate and hand tremors by a large percent. So much for relaxing!! So, our *rational* mind is not always correct, but, as long as our rational mind can come up with some reasoning for our actions, we will be at peace. Our *analytical* mind recognizes problems, such as a flat tire, and it figures out how to fix it.

Also, *will power* is in our Conscious Mind. How many times have you tried changing an old habit by using will power? Will power is only temporary. It gives us short bursts of energy to help us get through a mental situation, but then it fades away. Will power cannot affect internal change.

Change has to come from within our Subconscious Mind.

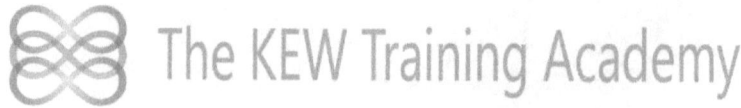The KEW Training Academy

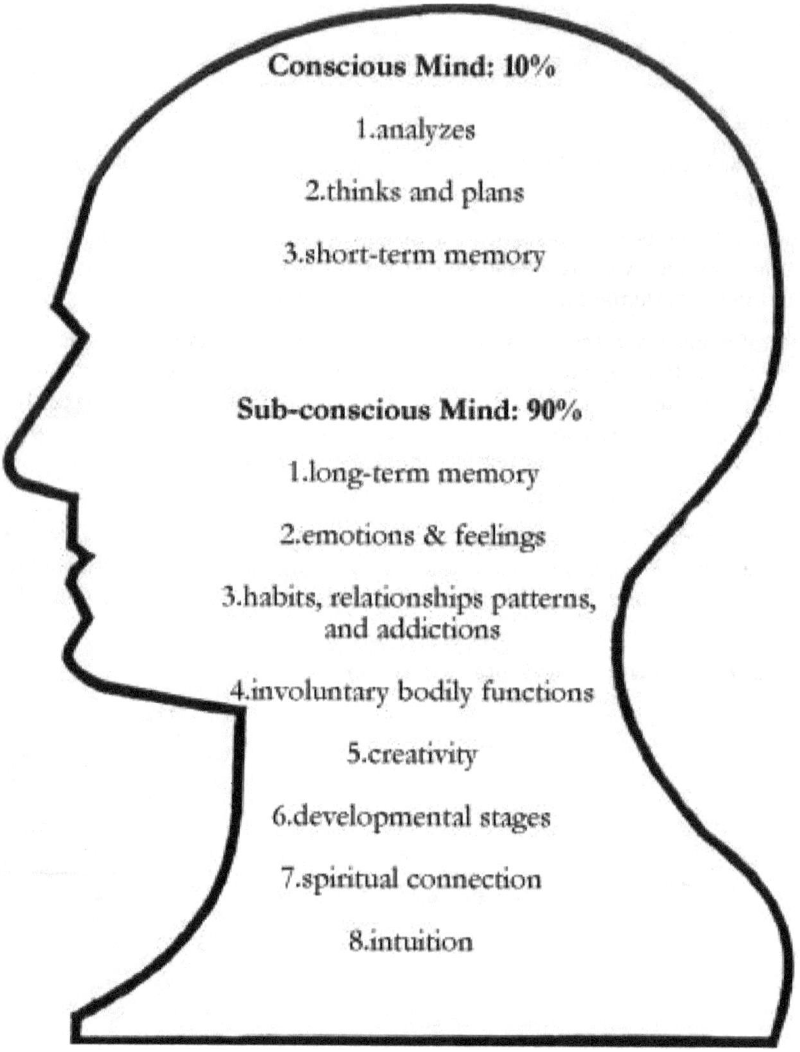

Conscious Mind: 10%

1.analyzes

2.thinks and plans

3.short-term memory

Sub-conscious Mind: 90%

1.long-term memory

2.emotions & feelings

3.habits, relationships patterns,
and addictions

4.involuntary bodily functions

5.creativity

6.developmental stages

7.spiritual connection

8.intuition

The fourth part of our Conscious Mind is our *temporary memory*. This is very limited. This is the memory that we need and use in our daily lives, like remembering where we live and people's names. Scientific research has proven that our Conscious Mind can only hold very small amounts of information at one time. And, this is the part of our mind that we use every day all day. Overall, the conscious mind is a very weak mind compared to the subconscious mind.

Hypnotherapy Practitioner Course - Professional Accredited Hypnotherapy Training

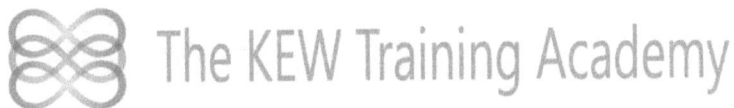
Subconscious Mind

Imagination, permanent memory, habits, feelings and **emotions, beliefs, Autonomic Nervous System**

The Subconscious Mind is the most powerful part of our mind. This is the part of our mind that is in control and that will help you to achieve your goals. The Subconscious Mind is the part of the mind that we work with in hypnosis; this is where our imagination is stored.

Imagination is more than just creativity. Imagination is also our perception of the world around us and everybody's perception is different. And, everybody's perception is the truth to them. Remember that perception is not reality; it's just a perception.

The Subconscious Mind is also home for our *permanent memory*. Every piece of data ever received through any of our five senses is stored in our Subconscious Mind. So, starting from when we were in the Womb everything we hear, feel, or experience leaves an imprint on us. Then we begin to build a database of information that develops into beliefs and habits, and all of this develops who we are today. We will think our next thought, act our next action, and feel our next feeling based upon everything that has happened in our past. We are the sum total of all our past.

Our permanent memory is like a hard drive on a computer, it is a highly organized system and we know that because it works by association. For example, if you are driving in your car and you hear an old song, feelings come back of some old friend or memory associated with that song.

Our Subconscious Mind is like our computer and sometimes we need to reprogramme our computers.

Habits, feelings, beliefs and emotions are also stored in the Subconscious Mind. The Subconscious Mind is the feeling mind. Hypnosis can help you become aware of the feeling or emotion that is connected to your issue. When you allow this to happen, you are on your way to making permanent change!

Our Autonomic Nervous System is things we know how to do automatically such as breathe, eat, our heart beat, and blood circulation. When we cut ourselves we don't have to tell ourselves to heal, we don't have to tell ourselves when we are tired or hungry, our subconscious part of the mind takes care of that for us.

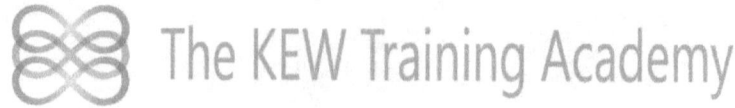

Understanding the Powerful Abilities of the Subconscious Mind

Here are some interesting mind teasers that will help you to understand the powerful and remarkable abilities of the subconscious mind.

Read the following paragraph and see how the mind seems to figure things out.

Your sucbsoncuois mnid is so fmialair wtih the wrods taht you raed taht it can roceiznge the wdros eevn if tehy are not sellepd coretcloy. As lnog as it has the bsacis scuh as the frist lteer and the lsat of the wrdos are there you can frugie out the rset on your own sicne wehn you raed you do not look at erevy ltteer.

When you read you do not read every single letter. You mind has the ability to skim over all the words and make an assessment of what it must be. This is usually done in speed reading.

Relax and concentrate on the 4 small dots in the middle of the following picture for about 30 seconds. Then close your eyes and tilt your head back slightly. You will see a circle of light developing.

Keep your eyes closed and you will see something emerging.

A hallucination? – What did you see?

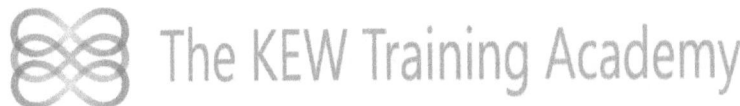
The KEW Training Academy

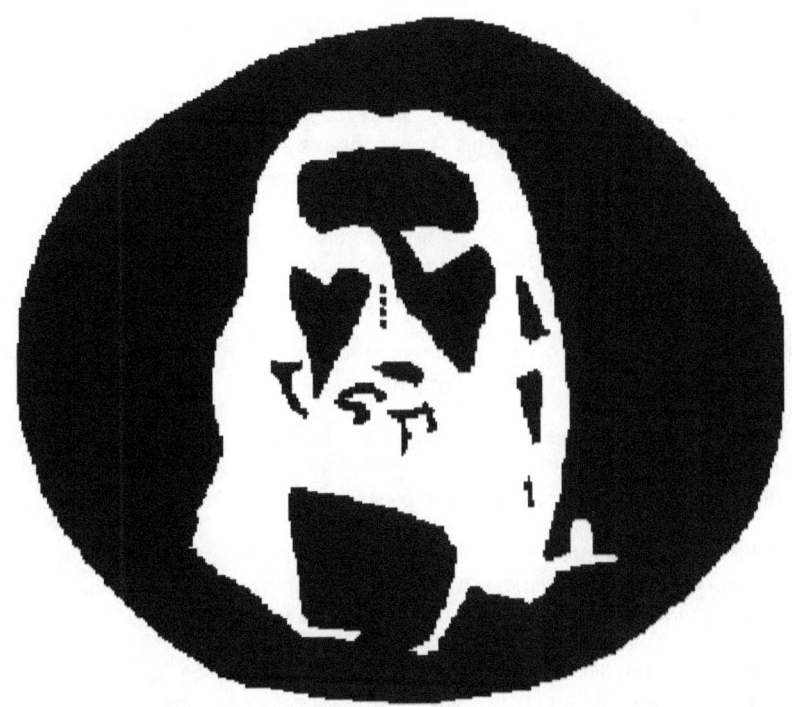

Read the following paragraph to yourself "once only" counting all the f's.

Finished files are the result of years of scientific study combined with the experience of many years.

How many f's did you find?

Only when you have finished the exercise read this below.

Read the above paragraph again and count the f's and notice the words of, now how many did you get?

The Great Hypnotherapist's of Our Time

Hypnosis has existed for as long as there have been human beings. This is because the hypnotic state is completely natural; something that can be achieved by everyone. Many ancient cultures have records indicating activity that might be described as hypnosis. Babylonians, Greeks, Egyptians, Druids, Vikings, Indian Yogis, Dervishes & Hindu Priests;

cultures using chants, drumming and dance rituals to change or alter the state of consciousness. These were often linked to religion or healing or both.

The earliest written records can be found in texts like the Ebers Papyrus; an Egyptian medical text dating around 1550BC. This scroll contains 700 'magical' formulas designed to cure afflictions ranging from crocodile bites to toenail pain. It also includes a surprisingly accurate description of the circulatory system, noting the existence of blood vessels throughout the body and the heart's function as centre of the blood supply. It contains a description of a physician placing hands on the heads of a patient and, claiming superhuman therapeutic powers, gave forth with strange remedial utterances which would lead to cures.

The Egyptians are also thought to have originated 'sleep temples' in which priests gave similar treatments through the use of suggestion.

Hypocrites discussed the phenomenon saying "the affliction suffered by the body, the soul sees quite well with the eyes shut". Among the Romans, Aesculapius often threw his patients into a "deep sleep" and allayed pain by stroking the patient with his hand.

In 2600BC the father of Chinese medicine, Wong Tai wrote about techniques that involved incantations and the passing of hands. Other accounts can be found in the Bible, the Talmud (a book of Jewish writings) and the Hindu Vedas, written about 1500BC.

The advent of Christianity led to a decline in the use of hypnosis because it was considered witchcraft. In the Religious Aspects of Hypnosis (1962) there are descriptions of how Jesus used hypnosis in performing many of his miracles.

Modern hypnosis started in the late 18th Century. A religious man called Father Gassner believed that patients who were ill were possessed by the devil. He performed a form of stage hypnosis. He told patients that when they were touched by his gold crucifix they would fall to the floor where they should await his instructions. They were told to "die" and an observer physician felt no pulse, heard no heart beat and pronounced the person dead. The demons were ordered to depart and then the patient revived. In the early 1770s this was observed by Mesmer.

Franz Anton Mesmer, (1734-1815), an Austrian physician, developed a theory called "animal magnetism," later named "mesmerism". He believed that disease developed when invisible magnetic fluids were cut off or improperly distributed due to the gravitational attraction of the planets. Mesmer believed that this mysterious fluid penetrates all bodies. This fluid allows one person to have a powerful, "magnetic" influence over another person. In 1775 he revised his theory of "animal gravitation" to one of "animal magnetism".

Mesmer used a tub filled with water and iron fillings, protruding from which were larger iron rods. He suggested to patients that as he touched them with his magnetic rod they would become magnetised and would eventually go into a state of "crisis" from which they would emerge cured. Many patients claimed that this treatment cured them.

He went to Paris to lecture and practice in 1778. His sessions, or séances, in which he supposedly "magnetised" patients, created a sensation. But the medical profession considered him a fraud. A French commission was formed to study the claims of Mesmer and his followers. It reported that the magnetic fluids did not exist. It explained the cures as a product of the patient's imagination. However, some of his patients and students continued to experiment with some of his methods and found that magnets and fluids were unnecessary.

Marquis de Puysegur, a follower of Mesmer, discovered a form of deep trance he called 'somnambulism'.

In the mid-nineteenth century a Scottish doctor, **James Braid**, pointed out that hypnosis was different to sleep and that hypnotism was a physiological response in the subject, not magical powers. He proceeded with experiments that disapproved the notion that the ability to induce hypnosis was connected with the magical passage of a fluid or other influence by the practitioner over the patient.

He had a psychological view that hypnosis is a kind of 'nervous sleep' induced by fatigue resulting from the intense concentration necessary for staring fixedly at a bright, inanimate object. He realised later that it was not 'sleep', but a concentration of the mind'. Perhaps Braid's most valuable contribution was his attempt to define hypnotism as a phenomenon that could be scientifically studied. Braid introduced the term hypnosis in his book Neurypnology in 1843. He later tried to re-name it 'monoideism', but 'hypnosis' already had strong roots in language. He was interested in the therapeutic possibilities reporting successes with paralysis, rheumatism and aphasia. He was also interested in aspects of panic and anxiety.

During this same period **James Esdaile**, a Scottish Doctor working in India, began to use hypnotism as an anaesthetic in major surgery, including leg amputations. He performed about 200 operations with the aid of hypnosis. As a result of his work the BMA reported in 1891, "as a therapeutic agent hypnotism is frequently effective in relieving pain, procuring sleep and alleviating many functional ailments".

John Elliotson, English physician who advocated the use of hypnosis in therapy and who in 1849 founded a mesmeric hospital. He was one of the first teachers in London to emphasise clinical lecturing and invented the stethoscope. Elliotson performed 1,834 operations using hypnotic trance. Elliotson also became an expert in child hypnosis too.

Jean Martin Charcot, a French neurologist performed landmark experiments in the late 1800s. He found that hypnosis relieved many nervous conditions. His clinic for nervous disorders achieved a widespread reputation among scientists of the time, including the French psychologist **Alfred Binet** and the Austrian physician **Sigmund Freud**.

Also in the late 1800's, the French physicians **Hippolyte Bernheim** and **Ambroise Auguste Liebeault** explored the role of suggestibility in hypnosis. These two scientists used hypnosis

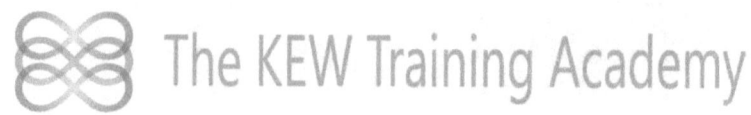

to treat more than 12,000 patients. Independently they wrote that hypnosis involved no physiological processes, but was a combination of psychologically medicated responses to suggestions.

Liebeault "the father of modern hypnotism", broadened the scope of hypnosis beyond pain control. He was adept at rapid hypnosis and he realised that a deep trance was not necessary, and he rarely spent more than fifteen minutes with his patients. He suggested away symptoms, "all phenomena in hypnosis are subjective in origin".

At this time a range of induction techniques were introduced. Liebeault was merely using the word "sleep" with a hand pass, Charcot on the other hand was violently ringing gongs and flashing drums lights. The Germans, Weinhold and Heidenhain, preferred the ticking of a watch, and Berger was using warm plates of metal. The idea of magnetism and magnetic processes had not yet completely worn off yet.

Despite Liebeault's explanation of the phenomena as subjective, Piteres maintained that certain portions of the body were particularly sensitive to stimulation of the skin, and these so- called hypnotic zones which were described by him existed sometimes on one side of the body and other times on both.

Moll has stated that he himself had seen many persons who were hypnotised only when their foreheads were touched. Purkinje and Spitt stated that touches on the forehead induced a sleepy state in many persons. Cradle rocking used to induce children was well known, and Eisenhart has mentioned stroking of the forehead as an excellent induction technique for children.

Hirt often used electricity to induce hypnosis, and Sperling, a contemporary of Bramwell's and Moll's, described the hypnotic trances of Dervishes which he had seen in Constantinople (now Istanbul).

Freud was especially interested in the work of Charcot and Bernheim. He used hypnotised people in his early studies of the unconscious state. He used it to help neurotics recall disturbing events that they had apparently forgotten. As he began to develop his system of psychoanalysis, theoretical considerations, as well as the difficulty he encountered hypnotising some patients led Freud to discarding hypnosis in favour of free association. However, he continued to view hypnosis as an important research phenomenon. Later in his life, Freud modified his once negative views on hypnotism.

Josef Breuer, Austrian physician and physiologist who was acknowledged by Sigmund Freud and others as the principal forerunner of psychoanalysis. Breuer found, in 1880, that he had relieved symptoms of hysteria in a patient, (called Anna O. in his case study), Bertha Pappenheim, after he had induced her to recall unpleasant past experiences under hypnosis.

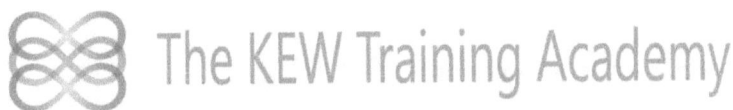

He cured a whole range of her problems by revealing more and more of her previous experiences. One was that she was unable to drink water; when she was regressed to the cause it was revealed that, at home, a dog had been given water from a glass; when she came out of hypnosis she immediately asked for and drank a glass of water.

In the 1880s, **Pierre Janet** identified the connection between academic psychology and the clinical treatment of mental illness. He stressed psychological factors in hypnosis and contributed to the modern concept of mental and emotional disorders involving anxiety, phobias and other abnormal behaviour. In 1891, the BMA reported favourably on the use of hypnosis in the field of medicine.

Various American scientists have made important advances in the study of hypnotism during the 1900's. Morton Prince showed that hypnotised people can maintain several mental activities at the same time. Clark L. Hull demonstrated that hypnosis is a form of heightened suggestibility.

Milton H. Erickson developed new strategies of hypnotism by combining clinical and research techniques. He was a master of indirect hypnosis; he was able to take someone into a trance without mentioning the word hypnosis.

Harold Crasilneck showed that hypnotic strategies can be effective with stroke patients. Herbert Spiegel described the natural hypnotic talents of patients. The studies of Ernest and Josephine Hilgard helped increase understanding of pain mechanisms in the body.

Hypnotism became widely used by physicians and psychologists during World War I and World War II. Hypnosis was used to treat battle fatigue and mental disorders resulting from war. After the wars, scientists found additional uses of hypnotism in clinical treatment.

In the 1950s both BMA and AMA issued statements supporting hypnosis.

Brain Waves and Functions

The human brain produces electrical activity that can be measured as brain waves. An electroencephalogram (EEG) measures brain waves in frequencies also known as cycles per second or hertz. Below explains four different brain wave states and how brain waves are related to hypnosis, the conscious, and subconscious minds.

Beta : Waking conscious state, alert 14-30 Hz

Alpha : Daydreaming, creative, relaxed, closed-eyed 8-13 Hz

Theta: Dreaming, hypnotic, meditative, subconscious, athletic "in the zone"

4-7 Hz

Delta: Unconscious, asleep, deep sleep 0.5-6 Hz

Hypnotherapy Practitioner Course - Professional Accredited Hypnotherapy Training

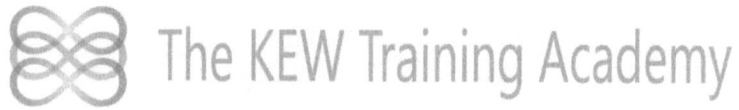

Beta Brain Waves

When you are awake, your brain waves are operating in the beta state of activity, that is, 14-30 hertz. Beta is the state of normal wakefulness. In Beta, you are alert and wide awake. Your conscious mind is dominant. This Beta state is where your brain waves would register during the beginning of your hypnosis session during the consultation process.

Alpha Brain Waves

When you close your eyes, become relaxed, or daydream, your brain waves are in alpha. This is the brain wave state of heightened creativity and inspiration.

When in the flow of being creative such as imagining or visualizing; your brains waves register in Alpha. In Alpha, your conscious mind is less dominant and the subconscious mind is coming to the forefront.

Alpha state is where your brain waves would register as when you go into a light trance (light hypnotic state). The subconscious mind does not register the difference between imaginary reality and physical reality. It simply does what it is told, shown, or imagined until it becomes a habit. That is why hypnotic suggestions can have powerful effects in the Alpha brain wave state.

Theta Brain Waves

When you are dreaming or in deeper hypnosis you are in Theta. Any repetitive movement or sounds will take you into the Theta state easily. This state is where much of your subconscious potential lies and where the subconscious mind is totally dominant.

Theta state is where your brain waves would register as your hypnotherapist takes you deeper into hypnosis where past experiences and emotions can be accessed so for example in a Regression session. In Theta, many people can go into deeper stages where also hypnoanaesthesia can be experienced.

Hypnoanaesthesia occurs when clients are so deeply relaxed that surgeries can occur with sensation but without pain. More people are using hypnoanaesthesia as an alternative to anaesthesia during childbirth, dental procedures, and surgeries since there is no danger of dying from hypnoanaesthesia as there is with anaesthesia.

Delta Brain Waves

When you fall asleep and go into unconsciousness, you are in Delta. In this state of consciousness, you will not remember what you are experiencing because you are asleep and will eventually go into the stage of deep sleep or total unconsciousness.

Delta state is where your brain waves would register if you fell asleep during your hypnosis session. Most clients do not fall asleep during hypnosis because that would go against the

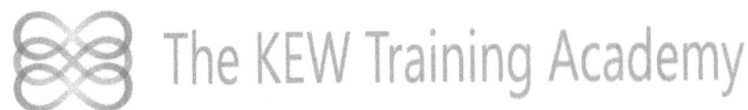

definition of hypnosis (hypnosis is focused attention combined with deep relaxation). If a client falls asleep during hypnosis, s/he has lost focus even though relaxation is deep. Clients may fall asleep for a brief moment or two, but normally, they come back into a Theta state where they can focus their attention.

Your brain can be functioning in more than one brain wave state simultaneously. For example, you can be in beta as you enter into alpha. You may be completely awake one moment and then feel more relaxed and close your eyes all in a few seconds. You could also be dreaming (theta) and rise up into wakefulness (beta) and then go back into a higher frequency (theta) than previously.

Understanding brain waves can help you connect the experience of hypnosis with brain wave activity in your brain. Most people enter Alpha and Theta states during hypnosis, and each subsequent time, they tend to go into deeper states of hypnosis or further into Theta. If you fall asleep during hypnosis, you have gone into Delta or deep sleep.

You are unconscious at this point, so suggestions cannot take hold in the subconscious mind. On the other end of the brain wave continuum, if you remain in beta, your conscious mind is dominant. You will have too many filters such as beliefs, values, ethics, and past conditioning to allow suggestions to take hold.

Processing information

Normally, the Conscious Mind can only handle 7 (plus or minus 2) chunks of information at any given time.

Try this: Can you name more than 7 products in a given product category, say cigarettes?

Most people will be able to name 2, maybe 3 products in a category of low interest and usually no more than 9 in a category of high interest. There is a reason for this. If we didn't actively delete information all the time, we'd end up with much too much information coming in.

In fact, you may have even heard that psychologists say that if we were simultaneously aware of all of the sensory information that was coming in, we'd go crazy. That's why we filter the information.

So, the question is, when two people have the same stimulus, why don't they have the same response? The answer is, because we delete, distort, and generalize the information from the outside. We delete, distort and generalize the information that comes in from our senses based on one of five filters.

The filters are, Meta Programs, belief systems, values, decisions, and memories.

"Behaviour is a mirror in which every one displays his own image" - *Johann Wolfgang von Goethe*

Hypnotherapy Practitioner Course - Professional Accredited Hypnotherapy Training

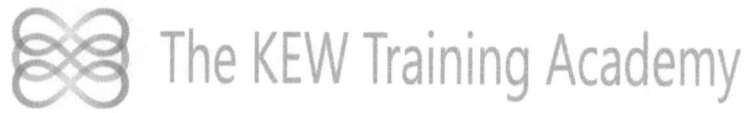

Behavioural traits are influenced by many factors that we will discuss later, the nature-nurture debate will always continue and who is to say who is right or wrong. One thing is for sure, there are key moments in our life that shape the person we become.

In the early stages of our life from the moment we are born and before in the Womb, the interaction we have with our parents and the closest people around us have a big impact and influence on us.

It's only after a few years that we also begin to model certain actions of the other people around us, parents, family, teachers, and our role models. How many people are inspired to go on and become a sports star, a musician, dancer, and a certain career path by being inspired by someone at an early age? Or as you become a parent yourself you find yourself saying the same thing to your children that your parents said to you.

Then as we get into our teens and beyond our social group begins to influence us, the people we socialize with have an impact on our lives. Their beliefs about the world, their aspirations, their social status all rub off on us and influence our behaviour.

The important factor is to separate the behaviour from the person. People aren't always behaving in one way all the time. People aren't always over eating; they don't smoke every minute of every day. People don't always react in the same way to certain events and situations. There are other factors involved in the thought process where the end result is a behaviour which we will discuss shortly in this chapter. Its relevance can be very powerful in helping us understand ourselves better.

Even within families siblings behaviour can be vastly different. I am sure we have all come across or at least read about families who adopt a set of behavioural patterns which see their lives shaped in a completely different way. Families of which one sibling becomes a successful business person, another turns to drugs or ends up in prison.

Let's take a moment to think...

Why do we do what we do, it is safe to say most people who smoke are well aware of the dangers of smoking, however carry on smoking. Most people know what foods to eat, that exercise is good for them. Let's explore and gain an understanding of why we do what we do, and by gaining that understanding we can change any negative patterns which aren't helping you live your life to the fullest.

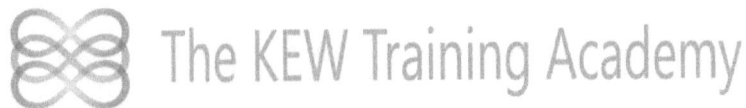

Perception

Complete the following exercise

What does the word relationship mean to you?

Now ask five different people what the word relationship means to them, and take note of their answers. Is every persons answer different?

Have you ever watched a programmed on TV then gone into work the next day and had a completely different perception of the programmed to that of your work colleagues?

If you had two different sets of fans watching a football match and the referee gave a close decision for a penalty to one team, would both sets of fans reactions be the same?

Why do people respond differently to different situations?

Have you ever heard the expression "that person lives in their own world" Well we all live in our own world which is unique to us and what forms that unique experience and influences our behaviors, our thoughts and our feelings.

The key factors are our filters, how we process information and interpret the information.

• Our Language • Memories • Attitudes • Values and beliefs • Meta programs • Time/space, matter • Energy

How do the above components influence our behaviour?

We have established we all make sense of the world in our own way. Our interpretations to events that are going on outside us are perceived differently from person to person, and as a result the behaviours that people manifest all vary.

First think about what is going through your mind at this present moment in time, this very second. Think about all the thoughts and feelings that are going through your mind this second. What are we aware of, the objects around us, our past, our future, our life, and the many thoughts which pass through our mind?

The things we stop and think about passing through our mind, what is for tea, have I put the bins out, I should make that phone call later, what's on TV tonight, I might go for a drive, and the list goes on. What are some of the things we notice and don't notice; different thoughts come into our mind at different times depending on what we focus on.

And at a conscious level we are limited to have many things we can focus on, let's explain:

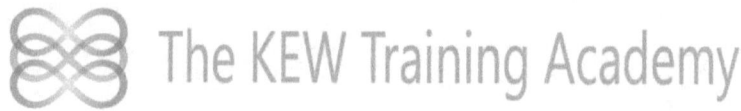

Our Conscious Awareness

It is estimated that your brain receives about four billion nerve impulses every second. Are you consciously aware of all of this information? No! For example, are you aware of how your feet feel on the floor? Unless you have sore feet I suspect that you were not aware of how your feet felt until I mentioned it. Why? Because it was not important at the time and it was filtered out.

Of the 4 billion bits of information, you are only consciously aware of about 2,000 bits, or about 0.00005% of all the potential information. To take in and process more of this information would either drive you crazy or be such a distraction that you could not function. Do you consciously remember every step you perform driving in to work in the morning, the traffic lights you stop at the gear changes. The people, the shops you drive past.

So of all the billions of nerve impulses our mind receives every second how do we interpret the information the way that we do? How and why do we all see things differently and what is the impact it can have on our life? How do we decide to interpret the information? What are the key components in breaking down this information to a manageable level in order for us to make sense out of it? Of the 4 billions nerve impulses that hit our mind every second, all of our past memories, and future plans, every event that is happening, all our interests, we filter, delete, distort, and generalize this information to the point we can make sense of it.

Filters - Deletions, Distortions and Generalizations

What happens to all of this other information? It is filtered from your conscious awareness by deleting (i.e. how your feet feel against the floor), distorting (i.e. simplifying) or generalizing. What you actually delete, distort and generalize depends on your Beliefs, Language, Decisions, Values, Memories, and Meta Programs.

For example your perception of a certain event can be completely different based on the part of the world that you live, your gender, your religion, your experiences, let us look at a few examples to gain an understanding of how they work.

Beliefs

Suppose you have a belief that you are unattractive or that you are not a clever person. How would you react when someone approaches you and says "You look very nice in that shirt or dress" "that was an intelligent point"?

Depending on the circumstances, you may dismiss, discount or deflect their positive feedback. Internally you may think they have not looked at it in detail and when they do they will find something wrong and change their opinion.

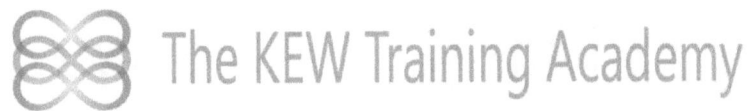

Suppose all day, people tell you that you're attractive or you're clever - do you really hear them? Not likely! And then one person points out that your nose looked a bit big on those holiday pictures, or the point you made at work last week was bit odd.

Does this resonate for you? You bet it does! It verifies your belief about yourself. From a 'filter' perspective, you have deleted and distorted the positive feedback and focused on the negative. What beliefs do you have about yourself, about others, about the world, that limit who you can be or what you can accomplish?

Language (Words)

Words are a form of code to represent your interpretation of something. Try this exercise, get a group of people together and have each independently write down five words that for them means 'exercise'.

I will bet that nobody comes up with the same five words as you do; and as a group you may not have any words in common. The word 'exercise' is code for what exercise means for you and I suspect that your friends have a completely different meaning for this word.

A perfect example are relationships, we enter into long and sometimes heated discussions with our loved ones about 'our relationship', without ever really discussing what 'relationship' means to each other.

Decisions

You make decisions (i.e. generalize) so that you do not have to relearn things every day. If you want make a cup of tea, you learned a long time ago (made the generalization) that you turn on the kettle, place a tea bag in the cup - you do not have to go through the whole process of relearning how to make a cup each and every time.

Generalizations are useful and they can also get us into trouble. How many of us know how to open a door, in an experiment, researchers put the doorknob on the same side of the door as the hinge. What do you think happened when they left adults in the room? They would go up to the door, grasp the doorknob, twist and then try to push or pull the door open.

Of course, it would not open. As a result, the adults decided that the door was locked and they were locked in the room! Young children, on the other hand, who had not yet made the generalization about the doorknob, simply walked up to the door and pushed on it and exited the room. The adults, because of their decisions, created a fear & reality of being locked in the room when in fact they were not.

So how many of your decision (generalizations) about yourself, your partner, your boss the way it is at work, leave you 'locked in', when others are not stopped by it? One of our challenges is to discover those filters I have put in place and how they affect what I see,

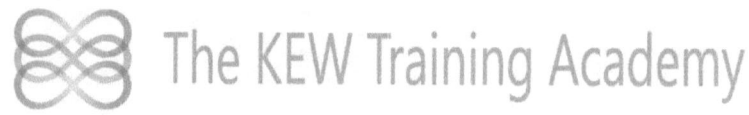

hear, feel; how I react to others and what I create in my life. Once you become aware of filters that do not serve you, you can choose consciously to modify or remove them.

Internal Representations

Do you remember when you first fell in love, do you remember driving in to work the other morning, and do you remember when you first passed your driving license? How do you remember it? Do you see a picture in your mind, or are there smells or tastes? Were there sounds - perhaps in your mind you can hear a radio? To remember an event, your mind uses pictures, sounds, feelings, tastes, smells and words.

These perceptions of your 'outside world' are called internal representations and are a function of your filters (i.e. beliefs and values). Your perceptions are what you consider to be 'real' or in other words your reality.

If you and I went out for dinner, our internal representations or perception of dinner will most likely be similar and different in some way - depending on what is important to each of us (our filters).

Dinner is not very controversial however, what about our views on a conflict i.e. war or political situation. Given our different backgrounds, we may perceive this very differently with significantly different reactions (behaviours).

Filters

Have you ever gone to see a movie with a friend, sat next to each other, saw exactly the same movie and one of you thought it was the best movie ever and the other thought it was terrible? How could that happen? It is quite simple. You and your friend filtered the information differently (different beliefs, values, decisions, etc.). In other words, you perceived the movie differently and hence behaved differently in your reaction to it.

By the way, who put your filters in place? You did! -- based on what happened in your family as you grew up, the teachings of your church (or absence of church), the beliefs and values in the part of the country where you lived, decisions you made about the world (i.e. a safe place or a dangerous place), etc. If your filters are not creating the results that you desire, you are the only person who can change them. The first step is to become consciously aware of the filters you have and what kind of reality (results) they are creating for you.

Internal Representations and Behaviour

Would you like to see the effect internal representations have on your behaviour? Can you think of a really happy event in your life? Close your eyes and get a picture of it in your mind, bring in any sounds, feelings, tastes and smells. Fully experience the event in your mind. Once you have done that, notice if there were any changes in your physiology. Maybe as a result of these memories (internal representations), you had a smile on the face, or sat up straighter, or maybe breathed deeper.

I am sure that your physiology changed in some way. I did not ask you to change your physiology, did I? What this demonstrates is that the pictures, sounds, etc. (internal representations) that you make in your mind, influence your physiology and as a result, your choice of words, the tone of voice you use and the behaviours you manifest.

Now sit up straight, put a big smile on your face, and breathe deeply. While you do that, feel sad. I will bet that you could not feel sad without changing your physiology (i.e. shallow breathing, rounded shoulders, etc.). This illustrates that your physiology influences your internal representations (feeling sad or happy). Next time you are feeling sad or down, what can you do? - Participate in some physical activity (i.e. brisk walk, exercise).

Based on your previous experiences, you filter information about the world around you. The resulting internal representations are how you perceive the world (your reality) and this drives your behaviours, often reinforcing that your perception of the world is 'correct'.

For me, one of the benefits of discovering the filters I have put in place and how they affect what I see, hear, feel; how I react to others and what I create in my life. Once you become aware of those filters that do not serve you, you can choose consciously to modify or remove them to help you take control of your life and creating a life you want, helping you break negative behaviours, un- productive thoughts, limiting beliefs.

Calibration

Calibration refers to the skill of observing and listening for the unconscious responses that our clients offer us.

These unconscious responses offer **clues** as to the thoughts that are passing through the mind of the other person. By noticing these clues, we gain insight that can help us to communicate with both the conscious and subconscious mind, and become more influential.

What is there to Calibrate?

Surely we are not suggesting that a client, just through normal conversation, will reveal her unconscious thoughts to us? Yes, she will and she does! We should firstly be aware that people reveal their unconscious thoughts when they are emotionally invested in what they are discussing. Often when people are discussing issues for the first time they can become more guarded, or more "consciously minded", or otherwise more difficult to read. Therefore it is easier to read unconscious response when we lead a person to become emotionally invested in what they are discussing. This means that we should ask questions such as:

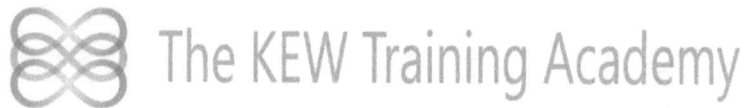

- What does this mean to you?

- Is this important to you?

- What will you get out of this?

When we ask questions that relate to how a situation will affect a person individually, we are much more likely to get unconscious response.

Unconscious Clues

So what would we be looking and listening for, to allow us to calibrate when we meet with a client? Here are some of the major clues that may reveal unconscious process:

Eye Movements

The way a person's eyes move can tell us what they are thinking. Essentially we tend to move our eyes a certain way, when we think in a certain way. By calibrating to how the person in front of us thinks, we can begin to recognize how they are thinking as we watch their eyes move.

Predicates

Predicates refers to the type of words that we use when we speak. In terms of Neuro Linguistic Programming (NLP), we theorize as follows: if a person says, "I see what you mean" it implies that they are seeing a picture. If they say, "That sounds right" then they are judging by hearing.

As we listen, really listen; to the words others use, we may begin to notice how they are thinking.

OTHER CLUES TO SENSORY PROCESSES

Several other clues can help us to understand how the other person is thinking. These clues may include:

• Breathing • Posture • Gestures • Voice tone • Speed of speech

Gestures

The gestures that a person uses indicate where they locate certain things in their map of the world. You will begin to notice that an individual consistently gestures a certain way when talking about a certain thing. This is not random gesturing; it has real meaning for that person.

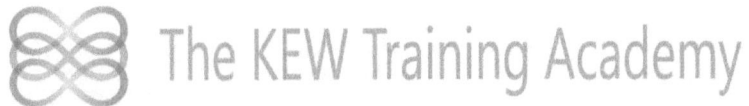

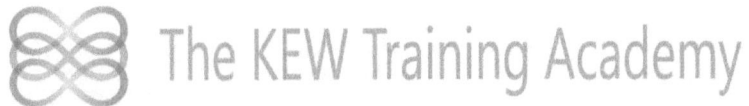The KEW Training Academy

Analogue Marking

People, whether in business or otherwise, tend to mark out words that are important to them. They may do so by, for example:

- Gesturing on certain words

- Adding additional tonal stress to a certain word

- Breathing at a different rate (or sighing) on a certain word

As an example, a student talks about a resourceful state that she felt. At the same time she makes a gesture by her side of rocking her hand, a universal signal for "I'm not sure". Noticing this we asked her if this was really the resourceful state she wanted to access, and she said no, there was a much better one.

The Map is not the Territory & Representational Systems

The map is not the territory is the idea that the way we represent the world refers to our own reality, it isn't reality itself. We don't respond to reality. We respond to our internalized map of reality. We all live in our own unique reality and we all see the world completely differently. We can look around and clearly see that we are all unique and different to look at but what we sometimes fail to realize is that we are all even more different in the way that we think and code the world around us. It is important to remember this when working with clients.

How we represent things are our interpretations. Interpretations may or may not be accurate.

All maps are inaccurate to some extent. A map of a street would need to be as large and detailed as a street to be accurate. A map is a summary of what we deem to be the important features.

Our language reveals the maps and models we use to guide our behaviour. Communication is how we explain the world to others and ourselves.

As human beings, we input output and process information about the territory around us. Our five sensory systems code this information.

Our five senses (visual, auditory, kinesthetic, olfactory and gustatory) are the language of our brain.

The NLP term for these five sensory systems **are representational systems.** When people communicate, they translate their experiences into words. Language is a representation of

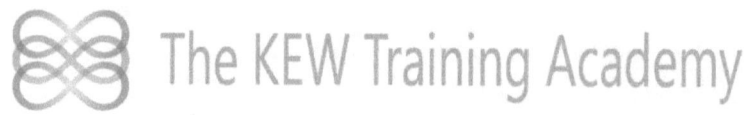

our sensory representations, a map of another map. Words have no built in meaning. Words only have meaning in that they trigger sensory representations in a speaker or listener.

As parts of NLP is modeled from Milton Erickson and Hypnosis there is a big cross over. It is VERY important to note down the language a client uses to describe their problem, this will give you the therapist an insight in to how they code the world around them and what representational system they favour most. Eg, Visual, Auditory, Kinesthetic, Olfactory, Gustatory.

Representational Systems

Representational Systems

There are five sensory channels we use to represent our experience - **visual**, **auditory** (hearing), **kinaesthetic** (emotions, touch and bodily sensations), **taste** and **smell**. In addition, we can make sense of our experience in words.

All of our memories, imagination and current experience are made up of elements of these six 'representational systems'. Most of us use one system more than the others. This shows up in the words that we use. These are often referred to as 'predicates' in the NLP jargon.

You can listen out for the dominant sensory words in what a person is saying and use words from the same representational system when you reply. If you use visual words to a 'visual' person, it's easier for them to understand because they don't have to translate from another system. This is another way to gain rapport, because you will sound more like the other person.

Different types of Hypnosis

There are two main styles of hypnotic communication; the **"authoritarian"** technique and the **"permissive"** technique.

The characteristics of each tend to differ and each tends to be more effective in different situations and with different clients. Often, however, the styles of communication will vary in the structure of the induction.

For example, the post hypnotic suggestions (suggestions given when the client is in a hypnotic state) are given in a more authoritarian style with some clients. Your observation of your client will determine how your will proceed. It is, therefore, vitally important that you observe your client in great detail and that you focus on listening to what the client is saying and how he or she is saying it.

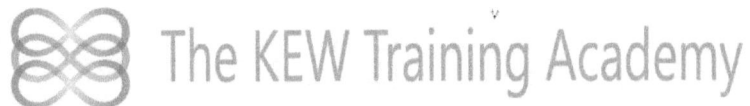
Authoritarian Style

This style of hypnotic communication tends to be direct and more commanding. The purpose envisaged with this style is to establish control over the client and, in doing so, give repeated commands to alter behaviour. It was thought that if the hypnotist exercised authority over the client it increased the chances of success.

The hypnotherapist tells the client what to do using authority and the client obeys. This requires personal power and authority from you the hypnotherapist. This style is best suited to subjects who are accustomed to and comfortable with taking instructions.

This style is successful when the client views the hypnotherapist as being an authority figure. The firm, direct commanding instructions convey confidence in the ability of the hypnotherapist and in the power of the induction. The heightened expectations very often increase the chances of success.

Permissive Style

This style of communication views the client as an equal partner in the hypnotic induction. More responsibility is given to the client. Imagery and a softer voice tone is needed to enhance suggestions. The Hypnotherapist suggests options to the client and gives the client the subject choice, or the illusion of choice. This involves cooperation between the hypnotherapist and the client. Success depends on language patterns skillfully used.

Direct

The hypnotherapist gives direct, clear instructions to the client and expects them to be carried out and acted upon exactly as instructed. The instructions are clear and direct but not necessarily said using a tone of authority.

Indirect

The hypnotherapist gives suggestions, uses metaphors, analogies, stories and ideas to intrigue the client. Hypnotic change happens as a result of the client's imagination being caught up and their subconscious mind responds to the ideas being suggested while the conscious mind is busy with something else. Milton Erickson favoured this form of Hypnosis.

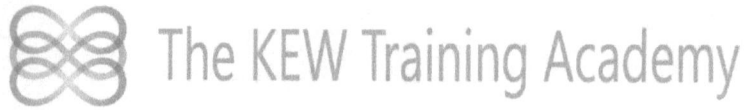
The KEW Training Academy

Theory about Types of Hypnotic Inductions

3 Distinctions about Hypnotic Inductions:

1. **APPROACH TO CLIENT: Authoritarian -vs.- Permissive**

2. **APPROACH TO TRANCE: Waking -vs.- Sleeping**

3. **APPROACH TO INDUCTION: Direct -vs.- Indirect**

Dave Elman had a completely different approach than his predecessors to the science of hypnosis. The types of inductions he utilised could be either: Authoritarian or Permissive, Waking or Sleeping, and Direct or Indirect!

His theory of hypnosis gave the client the responsibility for going into trance: "When a person rejects hypnosis, it simply means he has refused to *bypass his critical faculty* and [so has made] the *implanting of selective thinking* impossible. It doesn't mean he can't be hypnotized or won't be hypnotized, but simply that he refused to follow instructions. If he does follow properly given instructions, hypnosis is possible for him just as it is for everyone."

"Practically all textbooks declare that you must first obtain eye- closure if you wish to obtain hypnosis, and that eye-closure can usually be obtained by the methods called fixation, monotony, rhythm, imitation or levitation. I'll obtain eye closure without these methods. Close your eyes and pretend you can't open them. Keep on pretending, and while you are pretending, try to open your eyes. You'll find that it is impossible, if you are concentrating hard on the pretence. Now you know very well that you can open your eyes any time you change your mind and stop pretending. All the time you were pretending that you could not open your eyes, your sense of judgement was completely suspended concerning that particular action. You obtained the same eye closure you would if you used the techniques of fixation, monotony, rhythm, imitation or levitation. This can be done instantaneously.

Type of Hypnosis

Client

Trance

Induction

Traditional Hypnosis

Authoritarian

Direct

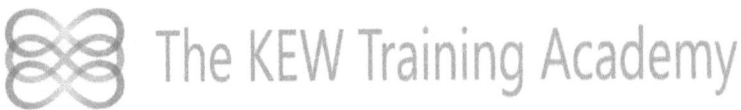

Ericksonian Hypnosis

Permissive

Waking

Indirect

NLP

Suggestion Therapy vs. Regression

Having looked briefly at Suggestion Therapy & Regression, it is important to understand the difference between the two. Both require inducing Hypnosis but as we have seen for Suggestion Therapy the Alpha state is acceptable and for Regression it is the Theta state required.

Suggestion Therapy is just that – Suggestion. You are making Suggestions to the Subconscious Mind to improve or resolve certain issues that are happening for your client. Most Hypnotherapist's use only Suggestion Therapy. If your client came to you with a Weight Problem and wanted to lose weight, once you had got to the Subconscious Mind then with Suggestion Therapy you would make suggestions that they would eat healthily, feel motivated to exercise and imagine themselves slimmer and fitter.

Regression simply means – going back in time. You can regress your client back to events in this lifetime or in Past Lives. However, Regression itself is a advanced form of Hypnotherapy and can be studied and performed once you feel confident and experienced with Suggestion therapy.

The Imagination

The Imagination is key to obtaining a depth deep enough for a Hypnotherapy session. You will need to find out from your client what their primary sense is: Are they visual; are they kinaesthetic, can they hear in visualisations? All are keys to a successful session. In the Induction, you will be describing various things to them, like a guided visualisation and you will need to know which of their senses are the most prominent. Only 50% of the population are visual, the other 50% are a mixture of sensing, feeling or hearing. This is going to be the same when they experience their memories. So, these senses link to the Imagination and if your client can imagine or sense what you are describing, you are halfway there to a successful session.

Clear & Clean Language

Clear and Clean Language is essential in Hypnotherapy. Clear & Clean Language starts from the moment that you come into contact with your client, by telephone, email and when they walk through your door. Clean Language is an excellent means of opening doors for the client and allowing the client to reveal the best choice of perception to themselves. In the Pre-Talk/Consultation, your client may talk negatively about an issue that they are dealing with, and during the Pre-Talk/Consultation you may re word this as something positive or put a spin on what they have actually said. In that way, you are getting your client to see things in a different perspective from how they see things now. It is always important to use only positive words that are going to help the client during Hypnosis rather than any of the negative things they may have mentioned to you.

A Focusing Of The Mind

All Hypnosis is Self Hypnosis which means the client is allowing themselves to go into that level of relaxation – The Hypnotic Trance. The Conscious Mind needs to focus so that the Subconscious can allow the memories (in Regression) to come up or the patterns of behaviour (Suggestion Therapy) to change. In the Focusing Of The Mind, you are using a Guided Visualisation (Induction) to allow the Conscious Mind to focus on the images or your words so that the gateway to the Subconscious is open.

The Safe Place

In your Pre-Talk/Consultation, it is a good idea to establish a Safe Place with your client. Again, this is just using imagery to evoke their memories. A Safe Place can be somewhere outside in nature that your client loves spending time at, or it can be a room in their home or really anywhere that appeals to them where they feel safe & comfortable. When they have told you the place, you then want to ask questions like: "What would the weather be like there for you on a perfect day?" "Would you be alone, or with anyone else?" Your client may say that their safe place is a white sandy beach, where they can walk across the sand, the sun is shining and it's warm but not too hot, there is a slight breeze, they can hear the crash of the waves from the sea on the beach etc. When you are in the Hypnosis session, you can bring all of what they have explained to you into the safe place and use THEIR words they have told you. So, again you are using imagery and their words to create the scene. If they are on the beach, they can walk across the sand – *feeling* (kinaesthetic) the sand beneath their feet, they can *hear* the crash of the waves (audio), they can see the white of the sand – *visual* – so you are evoking all of their senses and those senses become heightened.

Timing

Again, another important factor when it comes to Hypnosis is timing. Timing is somewhat of an art, especially when putting questions to your client and sitting back and giving them enough time to tell you what is happening and what they are experiencing in the session. It

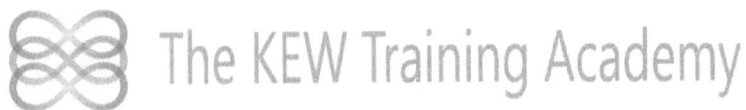

is a fine line of timing and compassion to ask questions and just sit back and let your client tell you in their own time what they are experiencing (See Abreactions) There is nothing wrong is sitting in silence for a few minutes while your client experiences what is happening in the session, it allows them to connect with what is happening at that time. This comes with a certain amount of experience from being a therapist but once you learn the art of timing, your sessions will become magical.

Deepeners

Deepeners and Deepening in and throughout a Hypnosis session is essential. Through the scripts you will be taking your client through different layers of deepening. Deepening just means taking them to another level of relaxation so they feel "deeper" in that relaxation that before. You will always hear Hypnotherapists say "going deeper and deeper" and that simple command is enough to take your client to that level. Deepeners can consist of just those words – "Deeper, feel yourself going deeper into a deep level of relaxation" or they can be imagery like a staircase with 20 steps – getting your client to imagine those steps and as you count the numbers backward in time – "20, 19, 18" etc they will be going into a deeper level of relaxation. The key as in all Hypnosis is **YOUR WORDS**.

Anchoring

Anchoring is an important part of any Hypnotherapy session. To anchor is to enhance the positive feelings that the client experiences during the session. So, if they are feeling joyful, strong, empowered or indeed any positive feeling, then you would anchor this feeling for them. To do this, you would simply get the client to breathe in the positive feeling and feel it move all the way through their body into every cell. Only anchor POSITIVE feelings for the client and never negative feelings.

The Return

As the session come to an end, it will be time to return the client back to full conscious awareness. You can say to your client the following: "I am going to count from 1-10, at the count of 10 you will be back here with me in this room, on this time, on this day. 1, 2 and 3, letting any scenes, feeling emotions, fade into the background, 4, 5 and 6, feeling yourself return to this room and moving fingers and toes, 7, 8, 9 nearly there, and 10 – whenever you are ready, opening your eyes, feeling safe, calm and comfortable, being grounded and right back here with me in this room now".

Give your client all the time they need to bring themselves back to full conscious awareness. Never rush the client returning. And remember, because they have been in a level of relaxation, a slight shift of consciousness, they will open their eyes and come back to awareness. It is impossible to "get stuck" – they will be right back with you in that room.

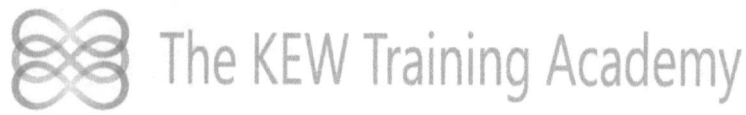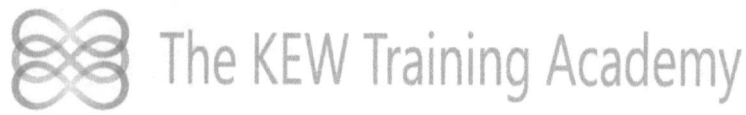The KEW Training Academy

Structuring a Successful Appointment

1. If a client calls to enquire about booking a session, you need to get as much information as possible from the client about their problem and ask them about their main outcome for the sessions. Work within your own time scales and set an appointment for them to come and see you for the first session.

2. It is advisable to do research in to how much others in your area are charging for Hypnotherapy sessions (I usually recommend 4 sessions if a client wants to come for weight loss, one session every week for 4 weeks although every client is different, I charge £60 per session for a Hypnotherapy session. If it's a smoking cessation session I do 2 sessions and charge £150. Find out how much other's are charging in your area and charge accordingly.

3. You can choose to either email a questionnaire over to the client to get as much detail as possible from them about their problem or you can gain the information from the client in your consultation before the first session begins. If you do email the questionnaire over to the client, ask the client to kindly email the questionnaire back to you before their session begins, this gives you time to get some background information on the clients problem and will help you to plan your hypnotherapy session. It will also point out on the questionnaire if there are any other areas that may need to be addressed throughout the session, any underlying issues that may be contributing to the problem. Also email over confirmation of their appointment details. As you become more experienced, you may find that you just get the information from the client in their pre-talk/consultation rather than emailing it to them first.

On the next page is an example of a Consultation form to use with your clients. Note the details needed that you will discuss with your client in the pre-talk/consultation.

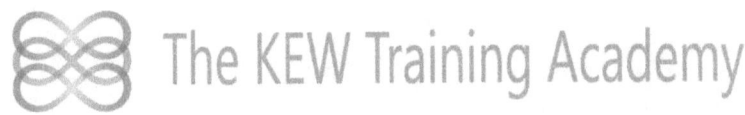
The KEW Training Academy

Full Name ....   Date...........................

Address...   Age............................

....   Married?........................

....   Children?.....................

Tel no...   Occupation.................

Email Address...

....

Are you currently taking any medication? ....

Have you ever had psychiatric treatment? ....

Have you any physical/medical condition?..

Have you recently gained or lost weight? ....

Have you recently consulted your doctor? ....

Tick all items that indicate a problem to you

Lack of confidence	Weight	Smoking
Insecurity	Appetite	Alcohol
Relationships	Nail biting	Grief
Unusual fears	Confusion	Guilt
Nervous symptoms	Sex	Worry
Stress/Pressure	Spiritual	Poor Sleep
Low Self-esteem	Blushing	Habits
Anxiety/Upsets	Phobia	Work
Eating disorder	Memory	Suicidal
Afraid to go out	Can't cope	No future
Skin condition	Pain	IBS
Jealousy	Anger	Self-harm

Other Problems ....

How many previous experiences have you had of hypnotherapy?...

Your Signature ....

Hypnotherapy Practitioner Course - Professional Accredited Hypnotherapy Training

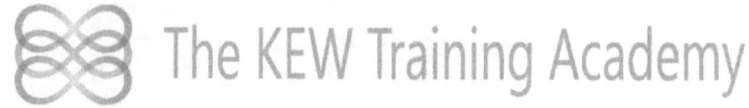

Contraindications

Special note should be given to the part on the form relating to previous psychiatric treatment and medication taking. You will need to check with your client about any episodes of previous psychiatric treatment and also any medication's your client is currently taking. You will need to know what the medication is for. Hypnosis is not recommended for anyone suffering from schizophrenia, psychosis or epilepsy. Be aware of your client's medication, they must not be under the influence of alcohol, drugs or anything related to the above conditions when experiencing Hypnosis. If in doubt, you can always ask your client to contact their General Doctor who must confirm to you they are suitable for Hypnosis.

If you choose to send the consultation form to the client beforehand, once received back you can then structure to how you want the first session to go.

Take a look at a Sample Weight Loss questionnaire on this page; this is from a client looking to lose weight. Read it very carefully and take note of what you find, are there any other issues that may also need addressing? Take note of the language used and the type of representational system used the most.

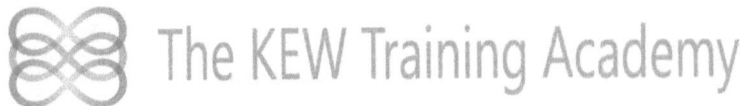

Sample Weight Loss Questionnaire

Name:...Laura ....

 Age:......38.................

Marital Status:...Single.

Occupation:......Accountant.............

Is your life stressful? Very!

If so, in what ways is it stressful............Work, Everyday Life Situations, Lack of Friends, Family Demands, I'm on my own ....

Partners name:............None.. **Age:**............N/A.......

Children:............None........ **Children's Names:**...............N/A.............................

How much weight do you want to lose?........56 1bs (4 Stone)..........

What is your main outcome for the session?........To enable me to eat healthy nutritious foods and to stop binge eating as its getting out of control and making me feel self-conscious and depressed ....

Why haven't you been able to achieve this so far?......I have been yo-yo dieting for years, and have been unsuccessful in maintaining the weight loss long- term. I have a very stressful life and assume the weight gain/binge eating is due to boredom, stress and loneliness ....

What particular type of foods do you want to stop eating?...Starchy foods such as bread, cereals and crackers...

Why do you eat these kinds of foods?....I do not cook, therefore these are convenience foods, quick and easy ....

Why do you want to stop eating them?.......I would like to eat more healthily and break the habit of binge eating when I'm down.............

How much of these foods do you tend to eat in a day?........Too Much , 6 slices toast, butter, jam, biscuits, all the wrong kinds of food ....

In a week?.................Every Evening

Hypnotherapy Practitioner Course - Professional Accredited Hypnotherapy Training

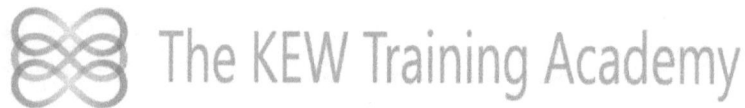

When do you tend to eat these kinds of foods? When I feel happy

When I feel down/sad/lonely **please specify**......................

When I'm bored/ tired

Other:...............When I feel down, sad, lonely and bored
....

What do you get from eating these foods? It gives me energy,It's a nice way to treat myself &I tend to snack when I'm bored. It gives me an energy rush &It gives me comfort & also relaxes me

Other:...

What time of day do you tend to eat these foods?

On waking, at breakfast ,with tea/coffee, after meals, driving

Other:...............At Home, I'm always alone

What frightens you about not stopping eating these foods?...............Becoming a Diabetic and Morbidly Obese ....

Do you know someone who has died from a weight related disease, or has any insulin related illnesses?

Yes No Yes

If so who? My Mother has an insulin related illness.....

What is your motivation for losing weight? Feeling More Confident , looking better, clothes fitting me better, getting into size 12 jeans, finding a partner....................

Who are you important to? My mum, family, sister Laura

Why?.........They love me, I have been single for the last 12 years, I'm very lonely.........

Has your doctor mentioned your over eating? Yes No

Have you ever had any worrying symptoms? Yes No

Do you have any health problems? Nervous Asthma and Depression

How long do you want to live?............a long healthy life

Hypnotherapy Practitioner Course - Professional Accredited Hypnotherapy Training

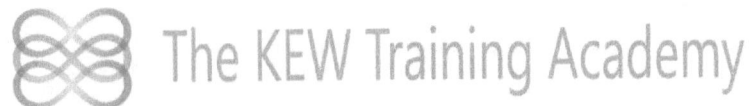
Why?................to have children and see them grow up

Who is responsible for your health?...............Myself

What will you be able to do as a slimmer healthier person that you could not do before?......With improved self-esteem hopefully I will have a positive outlook in my life in general and feel much better about myself...

What will you do with the money that you save?........Treat myself to some bright colourful clothes as I always wear black

Do you exercise at the moment?........I attend a Rosemary Conley Class twice a week

What forms of exercise do you enjoy?.........Walking and Keep Fit Classes

Do you really wish to commit yourself to stopping eating bad foods? Yes!

What is stopping you then?.....My Mother is constantly criticizing and telling me what to eat and what not to eat which makes me more unhappy ....

Do you have a goal, event or holiday coming up in the future that you would like to lose weight for? If so what exactly? I have a two week holiday booked to Corfu later in the year with my Mother

Are you 100% committed to stopping today? Yes!

Signed...... Laura...............................**Date:**...03/06/08...

What themes did you notice after reading through the weight loss questionnaire? Are there any other underlying issues that need to be addressed? In most instances when a client comes to see you for a session to lose weight there are usually other aspects involved. We all eat for different reasons, gone are the days when we all listened to our own inner hunger and only ate when we were hungry and stopped when we were full, in a lot of cases people tend to eat to feed an emotion, through habit or conditioned responses, we will look in to this more throughout the course in the weight loss section.

The purpose of the questionnaire is to take note of any specific language used (e.g. metaphors, analogies, types of words used, feelings, visual, auditory), to try and find the reasons behind their eating, what is over eating giving them, to get an insight in to the clients mind and how they are feeling, to find out if they on any medication or have any underlying illnesses and also to take note of everything that is important to them and everything that worries them about not losing weight. All the information gathered will then be used in the hypnotherapy session with the client. It is very important to try and use the clients own words and language throughout the hypnotherapy session when describing how they want their outcome to be.

Hypnotherapy Practitioner Course - Professional Accredited Hypnotherapy Training

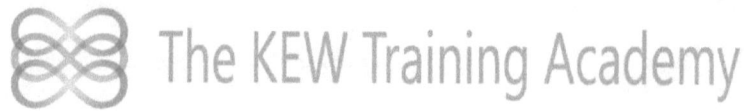
Key Points to Structuring a Hypnotherapy Session

1. Pre-talk/Consultation – this is gathering as much information from the client about their problem and *building rapport* with the client throughout, helping them to feel relaxed and comfortable. Identify any issues/problems the client has been experiencing (if any) that they want to resolve and prioritize the issues for you to work on.

2. Suggestibility Test

3. Induce Hypnotic Trance (Induction)

4. Deepen The Trance (Deepener)

5. Necessary therapy relevant to the client

6. Implant any post hypnotic suggestions

7. Awaken client from trance

Building Rapport with Clients

Rapport is the ability to relate to others in a way that creates a climate of trust and understanding. It is the ability to see the other's point of view and get them to understand yours. You don't have to agree with their point of view or even like it. It makes any form of communication easier and helps your client to relax.

Successful interactions depend largely on our ability to establish and maintain rapport. Surprisingly, we make most business decisions based on rapport rather than technical merit. You are more likely to buy from, agree with, or support someone you can relate to than someone you can't.

Rapport techniques are quite subtle but extremely powerful in their implications and effects.
Dictionaries define rapport as a relationship marked by harmony, conformity, accord or affinity. It supports agreement, alignment, likeness or similarity.

Emphasizing similarities

There are two ways to see other people. You can choose to emphasize the differences or the similarities between you. You can always find things you have in common with someone, even if it is just being human. Likewise, there will always be differences between you and another.

Even clones would have different experiences. If you emphasize the differences, you will find it hard to establish rapport. By emphasizing commonalities, resistance and antagonism will generally disappear, and cooperation will improve. With practice, it becomes easy to find what we share with other people and focus on it.

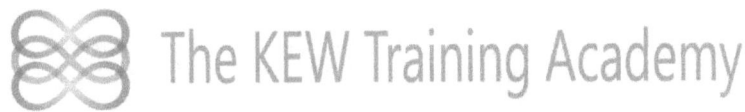

Pacing

Rapport can be established and maintained by pacing. By definition, this is the process of moving as the other person moves. Pacing or matching accepts the other person's behaviour and meets them in their model of the world. It is about reducing the differences between yourself and others at an unconscious level.

You can pace or match many different aspects of behaviour. Of course, if the other person is aware you are matching their behaviour it becomes mimicry. Obvious attempts to "copy" people will break rapport.

Successful pacing is at an unconscious level. When rapport is established, you can influence the other person's behaviour. If you would like to know if you have rapport, you can make a movement and find out if they follow you. For instance, you might scratch your nose and see if the other person does the same.

What you can match

Matching is something we all do naturally in some contexts. Watch what happens when someone talks to a small child. They might crouch down to the child's height, talk more slowly (or excitedly). Romantic couples in restaurants often seem to be engaged in a dance, leaning and smiling in mirror postures.

Body postures

You can adjust your whole body, half body or part of your body to match the other. Matching typical poses that the other person offers with their head and shoulders is useful. If the body posture is unusual however, matching can seem disrespectful. Subtlety is vital.

Breathing

A fantastic aspect of rapport building to master as it is totally out of the conscious awareness of the other person. You can match the rate of a person's breathing, where they are breathing (chest, abdomen or stomach) or how deep. This is not a good technique if the person has difficulty with breathing, as you may feel similar symptoms.

Voice

Matching the pace, volume, pitch, tone and type of words is a little tricky to learn but worth it. Try watching a TV program in a foreign language in order to notice these auditory processing distinctions. You don't have to try to match all these aspects. Choose one. If a person is talking slowly, slow down. If they speak softly, drop your volume.

Beliefs and values

Authentically trying to understand another person's beliefs and values without judgment can create very deep rapport. Once again, you do not have to agree with them or change any of your own values; the goal is to understand.

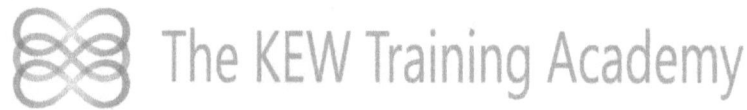

Language patterns

Matching language patterns is a favourite rapport technique with sales and marketing people. By using the same words to describe things and processes, the person feels understood.

Listen for their power words. We've often learned to paraphrase what someone says rather than use the same words. We call it active listening. This is mistake when it comes to NLP rapport. We attach particular words to corresponding experiences. If someone says she wants to be confident and you talk about her capability, you can miss the rapport boat.

Structuring a Successful Pre-talk/Consultation

1. Go through the questionnaire; let the client tell you in their own words more about their problem. Write down key phrases and words that they use to describe their problem these will be used later in the session.

2. Explain a bit about Hypnotherapy, dispel any myths and anything they might have seen on TV for example Stage hypnosis.

3. Explain the parts of the mind and how it works and the power of Hypnotherapy.

Ask them are they definitely sure that they are committed to changing today. On a scale of 1 to 10 (with 1 being not committed at all and 10 being definitely committed) how committed are you to changing today? If the client is less than a 10 on the scale ask them what would need to happen in order for them to be a 10?

Pre- Talk Information

During a pre-talk with a client it is very important to write down any key words or phrases that the client uses to describe their problem and situation. Clients will very often give you the answer to their own problems using metaphors, analogies and stories. If this happens it is very useful to write down the metaphor or story used and to relay it back to the client during hypnosis using the metaphor to form part of the solution.

For example:

A client may describe their problem in many ways, they may say that they "Feel like they've come up against a large brick wall and they just can't seem to get over it" or that they "have come up against a large mountain" or "that they feel like they are just treading water"

It can be useful to use the example metaphors that the client gives and use them in the session offering a solution.

For example:

Imagine getting a hammer and knocking the wall down... Imagine finding a door in the wall and simply going through it to the other side....

Famed Hypnotherapist Milton Erickson was a master at getting in to his clients mind using a form of indirect Hypnosis – metaphors, stories and analogies.

It helps the client to connect more with what you are saying and helps to build rapport speaking in the client's language.

Common Misconceptions about Hypnosis

Hypnosis is NOT Sleep

Your clients need to understand that they will not necessarily feel hypnotized, they will stay completely aware of things and sounds around them and they will certainly not be asleep.

You Will NOT Lose Control

It is a common held belief that a hypnotist exerts some sort of control over his subject, this comes from stage hypnosis and the old movies of Svengali type characters controlling the minds of others. Reassure the client that they are in control and at any time could bring themselves out of hypnosis.

You Will NOT Reveal Your Deepest Darkest Secrets

Again you are in control; you will only do and follow the instruction that morally fit for you. If there are things that you don't want others to know then you will in no way feel compelled to share these.

Being Hypnotized does NOT Mean You Are Gullible or Stupid

There is evidence to suggest that there is indeed a correlation between a person's level of intelligence and their level of suggestibility and it would appear that the opposite holds true, the more intelligent that you the more suggestible that you are hence the better a hypnotic subject you will make.

You Will NOT Get Stuck in Hypnosis

Very occasionally a client will not respond immediately to your requests for them to emerge from hypnosis, this is purely because the trance state is so relaxing and such a pleasant place to be that they are reluctant to come out.

Suggestibility Tests

Every person is a potential hypnotic subject, however, no one can be hypnotised without their knowledge or consent. By use of words and actions the hypnotist creates an illusion and if the person to be hypnotised is a willing subject, a 90% success rate can be achieved.

What makes a good hypnotic subject? It's not easy to look at someone and say whether they will be easily hypnotized or not nor are there certain guidelines that you can pick out in conversation that may help you to decide this.

There are, however, several tests that you can do that can indicate how receptive and responsive your client might be. These are called suggestibility tests. They are designed to see the suggestibility of the client, the greater the suggestibility, the more receptive the client will be.

Those that are more suggestible will be the easiest to hypnotise, those that are not may need a longer induction and deepener. These tests are usually carried out after your pre-talk

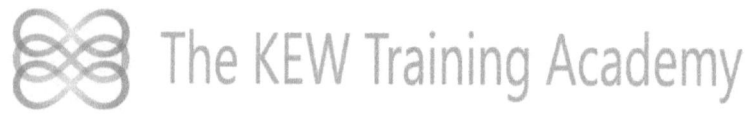
then a trance state can often quite naturally follow, as the tests themselves are hypnotic in nature.

In the following section you have three suggestibility tests you can use with clients:

Balloon and Book Hand Clasp Exercise Cheek or Chin

Balloon and Book

(First of all find out whether your subject is left or right handed. The following wording tells you what to say to a right handed person, but this should be reversed with someone who is left handed).

"Hold both arms out so that they are level and turn your left hand so that the palm is facing upwards, and the right hand so that the palm is facing downwards. Good, now check to make sure that those hands are level.

Now close your eyes and settle back into your seat and make yourself comfortable, because I'm going to test the power of your imagination and show you how your wonderful subconscious mind can work for you.

Okay I want you to imagine now that I'm placing on your left hand a very heavy book. The pages are very thin so there are literally thousands of pages which makes this book extremely heavy and you can feel it weighing down your hand.

And your hand is feeling heavy, it's such a strain holding that book - but wait, I'm going to place another book on top of that one; this book is a dictionary with a shiny cover and just as thick and just as heavy as the first - and your hand is getting really tired now - really, really tired and heavy - so heavy it just wants to go down - and down.

Your hand is getting heavier and heavier holding those books - it's going down and down and down and you're feeling more tired each moment from holding those books. But I'm going to place one more book and this time your hand will go all the way down. Just feel those books weighing you down - another heavy volume there on top of the other two and your hand is so tired - so tired - so tired".

(By this time you should have observed your clients hand going down, if it hasn't then continue in this way until it does, even if just a little).

"Good, now I want you to imagine that I'm tying a piece of string around your right hand and that the other end of the string is attached to a beautiful, brightly coloured helium balloon. The balloon is shiny and metallic on one side and it bulges out because it's filled with helium, making it lighter than air - so light that it floats right up, into the air - higher and higher - and as it goes higher and higher you can feel your hand lifting - rising — elevating, going higher and higher - feeling light and floaty as it begins to move upwards. The string holding the balloon is tugging at your hand - lifting it - raising it - higher and higher - higher and higher - floating all the way up - that's right.

Either ... (as a test)

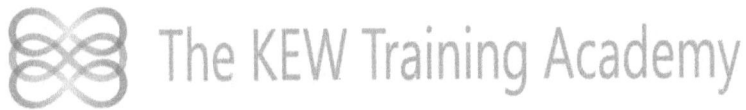

Alright that's fine, now open your eyes and look at those hands. (By this time one hand will be down on the lap and the other up in the air). That proves how powerful your imagination is and that you're going to be a wonderful hypnotic subject.

Or...(as a prelude to an induction)

Continue with another suggestibility test or an induction to induce trance (after instructing your client to let both of the hands rest comfortably in the lap and return to normality.

The Hand Clasp Exercise

"Make sure you are completely comfortable standing. Stretch your legs and arms. And begin to relax. Close your eyes and take a deep breath...and exhale...and relax. Completely relax. Relax your legs, lower back, relax your shoulders. Relax your shoulders, your arms, your neck, your face. Relax your whole body, just relax. Take another deep breath...and exhale...let go, and relax. Become aware of the rhythm of your breathing, and as you inhale, relax your breathing and begin to feel your body drift and float into relaxation. The sounds around you are unimportant, let them go, and relax. Let every muscle in your body completely relax from the top of your head to the tips of your toes. As you inhale gently, relax. As you exhale, release any tension, any stress from any part of your body, mind and thoughts."

"Clasp your hand in front of you and tightly push them together. Push them together very tightly. As you hold them tightly, imagine that a very strong, strong glue has been spread on your hands and glue is drying and keeping your hands together, your hands are tight together. Your hands no longer feel as if they are two separate hands. They are one. Your fingers and palms are glued together, hard and fast, very hard and fast. You test to see how strongly the glue is holding your hands, and you find your hands, the palms of your hands, your fingers are stuck together. They are stuck together.

They are glued together so tightly they feel as one. They are glued together very, very tightly and feel as one. On the count of three you will be able to pull your hands apart. The harder you try to pull the apart, the more they will stick together. They will stick together more each time you hear a number. One ...two...three.

Now I will count from five to one. When I say five you will begin to relax your hands as they start to return to normal – the glue no longer exists. As you hear each number you will relax your hands more and more, then when I say one your hands will be completely relaxed at your sides. Five...beginning to relax each hand...four...feel your hands relax...three...two...and one...your hands are completely relaxed and feeling normal to you."

The degree to which the client responds freely and easily indicates his/her suggestibility. Suggestibility exercises measure receptivity and responsiveness to suggestions. The greater the clients suggestibility, the more receptive a hypnotic candidate the person will be. However do bear in mind that this doesn't guarantee total success.

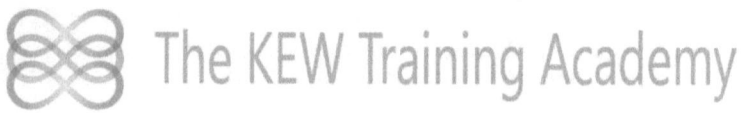
Cheek or Chin

This suggestibility test can be used to determine whether a subject has a visual or auditory representation system, which can help you to determine the pattern of induction to follow. It's also a wonderful icebreaker and pre-induction for children.

Whilst sitting opposite your subject, using your index finger and the middle finger and a raised thumb, say to your subject:

'Make a gun with the thumb raised' (show them the gun).

'Now - with your thumb and index finger - make a circle'.

When your subject has done this to your satisfaction, tell them: -

'Now - concentrate on the circle'.

Then say to your subject - 'Now place the circle on your chin' **(Whilst you place the circle on your cheek - notice whether he or she is placing the circle on the chin or the cheek).**

As the subject is watching what you are doing they are most likely to follow your movement and touch their own cheek. Draw their attention to it - 'Why are you touching your cheek?'.

If they follow your own movement, explain that this means that they are likely to be a good subject - if they don't follow your movement explain to them that are using their auditory representational system and remember, whilst hypnotizing this person, he or she is probably not as visual as most subjects. For clients who successfully copied your movements, follow this suggestibility test with another one, balloon and book and then a deepener.

Five conditions the hypnotic state will bring about in a client are:

- Body and mind relaxation
- Focus of attention
- Reduced awareness of external environment
- Greater awareness of internal sensations
- A trance state

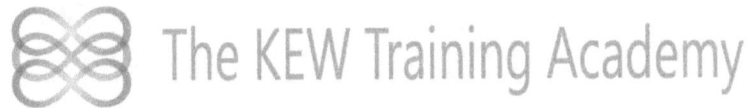
The KEW Training Academy

Induction Techniques

The Structure of an Induction

Before you design, compile and write an induction, it is very important that you know the structure of an induction, irrespective of the kind of induction.

Step 1: Beginning the induction

"Take a nice deep breath, close your eyes, and begin to relax. Just think about relaxing every muscle in your body..."

As your client begins to focus on their breathing and inner sensations, awareness of external surroundings will decrease. By breathing deeply, the client becomes aware of their internal sensations. The body is introduced to relaxation. The results are that the pulse slows, breathing slows, the client begins to withdraw and they can direct attention to the suggestions that are given.

Step 2: Systematic relaxation of the body

"And begin by letting all the muscles in your face relax, especially your jaw;; let your teeth part just a little bit and relax this..."

As your client concentrates on relaxing, they will experience an increased awareness of internal functions and an increased receptivity of the senses.

Step 3: Creating imagery of deeper relaxation

"Drift and float into a deeper level of total relaxation. Feel a heavy, heavy weight being lifted off your shoulders....."

The image of drifting down deeper and deeper helps to enter a deeper trance. The tension in shoulders is released as the "weight" is lifted from the shoulders. Any difference in bodily sensations will support the suggestions that a change is taking place.

To create a feeling of lightness, the following image could be used.

"You are feeling lighter and lighter, floating up higher and higher into a comfortable state of relaxation."

The direction, upward or downward, specified in the induction does not matter as long as it makes it possible to experience a change in physical feelings.

Step 4: Deepening the trance

"Imagine a beautiful staircase. There are ten steps, and the ten steps lead you to a special and peaceful beautiful place. I'm going to count backward from ten to one, and you can imagine taking the steps down and, as you take each step, and relax even deeper, 10, relax even deeper, 9 more relaxed, 8, 7, 6, 5, 4, 3 deeper relaxed, 2 more relaxed, 1 deeper and deeper."

In order to further deepen the trance state a count is used that usually goes from ten to one. You count backwards from ten to one as a trance deepens and forwards from one to ten as you return to full consciousness.

Hypnotherapy Practitioner Course - Professional Accredited Hypnotherapy Training

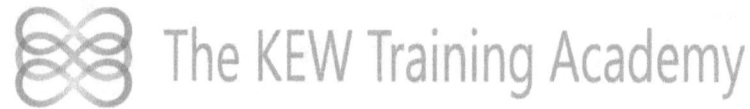
Although the image of a staircase was used above, you can substitute any image you like in order to enhance the feeling of going down. You may want to use the image of an elevator descending ten floors, as follows:

"You are in an elevator and feel yourself begin to descend. As you watch the numbers of the floors passing, you see the number ten...and now the stiffness of the limbs will occur. Attention will have narrowed and suggestibility heightens. You will also experience an intensification of the creative process."

Step 5: The special place

*"And now imagine a peaceful and special place. You can imagine this special place or perhaps you can even feel it. You are in (*insert description of special place). *You are alone, there is no one to disturb you. This is the most peaceful place in the world for you."*

The special place chosen will be one that is unique to the client and their experience. It can be a place actually visited or one that is imagined. The place does not have to be real, or even *possible*. It can be in a cave or clouds. The special place must be one in which the client can be alone and it must produce a positive feeling in you.

It is in this place that they will have an increased receptivity to further suggestion.

That is, once a peaceful feeling is established, the client will be responsive to imagery that reinforces and supports posthypnotic suggestion.

Step 6: Concluding the induction

"Enjoy your special place for another moment and then I will begin to count from one to ten and you can begin coming back to full consciousness, come back feeling refreshed as if you had a long rest. Begin to come back now. One...two...coming up, three...four...five...six...seven...eight...nine...and ten, open your eyes and come all the way back, feeling great. Very good."

Language Used In An Induction

The language of an induction is designed to communicate opinions, thoughts and feelings. It focuses attention on the client, their inner feelings and body. It also helps the client to become absorbed in their imagination and to communicate below the level of consciousness. Pay attention to the following components of language.

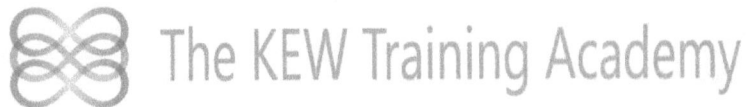
Synonyms

Instead of using only one descriptive word exclusively, synonyms are used for reinforcement when describing the desired state. They strengthen the suggestions. For example, "You are feeling at ease, relaxed, calm, and comfortable."

Paraphrased Suggestions

Suggestions are repeated and paraphrased to enhance comprehension and to ensure retention. For example, *"Feel the relaxation flow through your body, feel the warmth of relaxation, relaxing every muscle in your body, feel all the muscles in your body relax."*

Connective Words

Connective words have two functions; 1) to maintain steady flow so the monologue will not be interrupted and 2) to precede a directive, such as *"**and** now relax, feel all the muscles relax now **and** breathe deeply now **and** relax all the muscles in your arms **and** because you are relaxed feel a warmth flow through your body..."* In this context, the connective word *and* is a cue to respond.

Time Designations

Words that specify time are used for stress and emphasis. They can signal the time the suggestions begins of the time it ends. For example, any of the following cues could be used to signal the beginning of a suggestion: *"And **now at this very moment** release all tension from your body."* *"In just a few moments you will experience total relaxation."* *"In the morning **you will awake refreshed and relaxed."***

Eye Fixation Induction Script

Ok just make yourself comfortable and relax back into your seat and I want you to roll your eyes back and up as if your trying to look at your eyebrows, its important to feel your eyes straining just a little because looking up will give you a burst of alpha brain waves, so now go ahead and fix your eyes at a real or imagined spot on the ceiling and just keep your eyes glued to that spot and breathe in... and just breathe out.... keeping your eyes glued to that spot... and again breathe in... keep your eyes riveted to that spot... and breathe out... and just one more time breathe in... and just hold it and this time as you breathe out keep your eyeballs up but just close your eyelids right down.... and now that your eyelids are closing down just leave them closed and just allow a drifting floating feeling to develop in your body... don't try to make it happen... just let it happen.... just imagine a wave of deep relaxation washing over your body like water in the shower.... going from your head down to your toes .

And I want you to picture ten steps going down... and if your drop your chin just a little you can really get that looking down feeling that you get when you look down a flight of stairs... or out of an upper window... so get that looking down feeling right now... and as I count backwards from ten to one you can literally feel your feet moving onto step ten, you can see your feet making contact with step 9, you can hear your feet touching step 8 and now your taking step 7 and 6 and just going deeper into relaxation , your taking step 5 as each muscle turns loose, lets loose and you go deeper, your taking step three as you gently calmly easily move on to an even deeper level, your taking step 2 and now your taking the last step 1 and you are just going deeper and deeper and deeper into a comfortable, calm state of deep relaxation, and you can see everything, hear everything, feel everything and you are going to really like it , even when you are not aware of it your brilliant mind is seeing, believing and accepting every word I'm saying as you become more and more relaxed and calm.

And as you completely relax now both your mind and your body, I want you to focus on the word calm in your mind... and as you focus on this word, just allowing any stresses or strains from the day to just gently and easily start to drift away, no longer, needed, just taking this time for you today to completely relax and unwind....CAAAALM.... And as you step off the last step, you see in front of you a large door.....you walk over to the door and slowly go through......and as you go through you enter into your own special place of paradise, wherever that may be....somewhere you can go to totally relax and let go.....a special place for only you....where nothing matters.....no worries, no cares, you feel totally calm, safe and secure and you can enjoy the peace of mind, knowing nothing can bother or distract you, completely letting go now......CAAAALM.....and as you look around you....see what you see......hear what you here....and feel what you feel......engage all your senses and just completely relax....enjoying this time just for you..........

Ticking Clock Induction Script

Now that you're resting comfortably there....with your eyes closed..... feeling safe and secure...... I want you to take three very deep breaths and then breathe normally.... So go ahead now..... breathe in..... very deeply........ and now exhale...... Now take a second breath....... Inhale........ and exhale. And now........another.......inhale..........exhale..........Now be aware of your eyes...... how comfortable they feel ....closed........and just breathe normally. I want you to concentrate on only my voice now...... putting aside any other thoughts that come to mind....... And I'm going to draw attention to various parts of your body...........and as I draw your attention to that part........ then I want you to relax every muscle and nerve...... in that part of your body.

First of all I want to draw your attention to your fingers...........and your hands.........your wrists..........your forearms.........and your upper arms.........and as you consider this area of your body........I want you to be aware of any tension in those muscles........and concentrate on that tension. Now .....relax all those muscles..........every nerve ......every fibre.......in your hands and arms.......allow all of that tension to flow away.......to drain down.......let those muscles come to rest........lengthen and loosen......let them just feel very comfortable........heavy........very relaxed.......very........very relaxed.

And when you have relaxed those muscles in this way......then I want you to concentrate on your feet......your ankles.........your calves........your knees and your thighs.......be aware of any tension in those muscles.........and as you concentrate on them........then again........relax every muscle....... Every fibre in your legs and feet.........allowing all of that tension to flow away..........to drift down........lengthening.......loosening.......so that these muscles too feel very loose and comfortable.......heavy.......very.........very relaxed.

Now be aware of your stomach muscles........and your chest muscles.......and notice too how all the muscles in this part of your body are now becoming more and more relaxed......lengthening..........loosening..........much more relaxed......coming to rest as all of the tension just drains away.......draining away now just like the grains of fine sand in an hour glass drain down into the bottom of the glass. Now be aware of your shoulders......the muscles in your neck and your scalp......be aware of the tension here.......and now you can release that tension as every muscle in this part of your body now becomes more and more relaxed.......loosening and lengthening.......very..........very relaxed........so that you can feel all the muscles throughout your entire body now...... loose......limp and relaxed.........as that comfortable heaviness continues now.

And while your resting in this way..... I want you to imagine that it's a beautiful summers day.......I want you to imagine that you are floating on a cloud ....its so quiet and peaceful.......and there you are.......at ease with the world..........just drifting and dreaming as you float on and on and......on and on...... Now you're feeling very comfortable........so much at ease and completely relaxed.......and its such a pleasant feeling.....such a soothing feeling.......a feeling as though you just want to drift far far away......into a deep.......sound ......heavenly sleep.......You're so much at ease.......and every muscle and nerve in your entire body is completely relaxed and at ease.........and you feel so pleasantly heavy.........so completely relaxed.......that you just want to continue in this way........going into a deeper..... deeper relaxation.

Every part of your body feels so heavy and comfortable.........so easy......I wonder now if you can just let yourself sink and drift........deeper.......further into relaxation. And now I'm going to count from one to three.....and on the count of three......I want you to have drifted into a much ......much deeper relaxation than the one you are in right now.

One. And your entire body is completely relaxed.......every muscle and nerve is completely relaxed and at ease.......and your body feels so heavy.

Two. Your head feels so heavy and sleepy.......Such a very pleasant feeling......You feel so heavy and tired.......and you keep falling further and deeper into relaxation.......any your thoughts are vanishing.......All you can do is think of relaxation.....deep.......sound relaxation.

Three. You are now in a deep........sound relaxation.......and you'll continue to drift deeper and further......so that every word I utter will put you into a deeper and sounder sleep.......and all you can hear is my voice......You can hear no other sounds.......All the other sounds that surround us........Background noises.......traffic outside......all of these are insignificant......you become oblivious to all of these.......because all that is important is the sound of my voice.

Now (client's name)....... I want you to imagine there's a clock here in the room, and I want you to imagine the sound of that ticking clock, its steady relaxing ticking back........and forth.... Back....and forth.... As it marks time. The ticking of the clock that you are so aware of now.......is going to relax the rhythm of your brain......and as the rhythm of your brain slows down comfortably.........so then will you drift into a deeper........and deeper relaxation.

Now I'm going to count from one to seven......and I shall use the words "drift deeper".... In between each count......and you'll find that by the time I reach the count of seven.......you will be very....very deeply relaxed:
One....... Drift deeper
Two......drift deeper
Three....... Deeper and deeper...... drift deeper
Four ....drift deeper......
Five.........much much deeper into hypnosis.........drift deeper Six........Drift deeper Seven..........and now into a deep........satisfying and comfortable trance state.

And now I want you to notice that in a few moments......that you will no longer be aware of that ticking sound.... And when this noise stops.....that the rhythm of your brain will have slowed down to the extent that you will be aware of nothing....... Nothing but a beautiful silence......a complete silence......a peaceful silence..........in which nothing but the sound of my voice breaks through.

When this noise stops....... You'll be aware of only the sound of my voice........ no other sound will be of any consequence to you...... I want you now to enjoy that silence.......because with this silence....... You have achieved a peace that is yours....... Relaxation is yours....... And you can feel yourself in harmony with nature. You can now enjoy peace....... Tranquillity and a oneness with your own wise inner mind where all can be resolved and made good.

Continue with session... Deepener and Therapy Work/Technique

Induction Script - A Beautiful Day

Imagine yourself outside in your favourite place in nature. It could be a peaceful tropical beach, it could be a lovely old garden, or perhaps you could imagine lying back on a boat which is sailing on a beautiful river. It really doesn't matter where you are, as long as it feels good to you. Nod your head when you are thinking of somewhere special.

Good. And it's a beautiful day. The sky is a special shade of blue, very clear and its a warm day, a warm summer's day. And in the sky is a dazzling sun. It's so bright that you just want to close your eyes and feel the warmth of the sun on your body.

So imagine this now, in your mind. And surprisingly you find that you can direct that sun over and around your body, and as you realize this, you begin to direct the light from the sun over your face. And you can feel the warmth of the light from the sun on your face, just relaxing those muscles around the eyes and the nose and the mouth. And as you do this, you find that the facial muscles begin to flatten out as they relax, and you let go.

And it's a beautiful day. You move the light from the sun into the throat area, feeling the warmth of the light from the sun in your throat, relaxing all those muscles, letting go. And

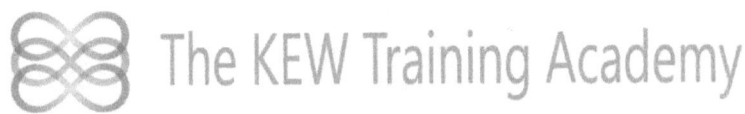

the sunlight moves into the shoulders and across the shoulders, making them feel loose and limp and comfortable.

You feel so relaxed, so comfortable and at peace with the world. And you direct the light from the sun down the right arm, from the shoulders to the tips of the fingers, the right arm begins to relax and let go, relax and let go. And it's a beautiful feeling to be here right now. The warmth of the light from the sun penetrates the nerves and bones and muscles of that right arm.

It is such a beautiful day. You move the sun over to the left arm and guide the light from the sun down and up the left arm, from the top of the shoulders all the way down to the tips of the fingers - you can feel the left arm relaxing, becoming heavy, and comfortable and relaxed.

Now move the light across and into the chest area and relax the chest and all the muscles there. That's good. Now the stomach, relax the tummy and down to the hips and the thighs and over to the right leg.

Relax the right leg. Let it feel really comfortable, let it relax. Now move the light from the sun down the right leg, up and down, from the top of the hips to the tips of the toes, and the right leg relaxes, and let go.

And it's a beautiful day. Move the light into the left leg now and move it up and down the left leg, from the top of the hips to the tips of the toes, and the left leg relaxes, releases all tension, let go.

You're whole body is now totally and completely relaxed, from the top of your head to the tips of your toes. And as your body relaxes so does you mind. And as your mind relaxes.. just notice the sun going down... going down and down... deeper and deeper. And the sky is ablaze with an abundance of colours of crimson... and bright purple... and blue yellow streaks. And it's a beautiful evening - your mind relaxes and lets go... releases all the stresses of the day... Let go.

And the sun goes further and further down, over the horizon, until, in it's place, is a black, velvet sky, and twinkling up there in the sky is a single twinkling star. Now keep your mind focused completely on that star. Nothing else matters except this beautiful single solitary sparkling star in the sky.

And it's a beautiful night. Apart from the start it is very dark, but you feel so safe, so comfortable, so relaxed, and at peace with the Universe.

Imagine yourself now, moving toward that star in the sky, moving up, and up and up. Your body is weightless as it lifts up to the star, going higher and higher, up and up. And as the star grows bigger and bigger you realize you're getting quite close to the star. It just gets bigger and bigger, brighter and brighter.

Until all at once you are that star in the night sky. That beautiful star, twinkling away, that silver solitary star in the night sky. You become the star and the star is you. You are one, back from where you came.

And it's a beautiful star. And as you just go deeper and deeper relaxed... Just let your mind go, let it wander just as it will. And as you simply relax...listening to the sound of my voice... I have some matters of great importance to say to you - and your subconscious mind will listen, accept and act upon the messages it hears. Everything that I say will become embedded in your subconscious mind, growing stronger and more powerful with every second....every minute...every hour....with every day that passes...helping you to move closer to achieving your goal."

(Carry on with session, use a deepener or continue with therapy work)

Eye Fixation and Arm Levitation Induction Script

For use with clients who expect, or are seeking a demonstration of Hypnosis. This approach helps to validate hypnosis as a real and potentially influential phenomenon.

"The first thing I would like you to do, before you continue to relax and enter into a relaxing trance, is to place the very tips of your finger tips very lightly on your thighs, with your arms in the air, elbows away from your sides, as if your arms and hands were just floating there, fingers just barely touching the material, so you can just feel the texture. That's right....

Fingers just barely touching, and focus your full attention on those sensations in the very tips of those fingers, where they just barely touch, where that floating continues, because, as I talk to you and you continue to relax, and to pay close attention, to those sensations.... I want you to look up at the ceiling...right up....and pick a spot there, anywhere at all....on that ceiling there...and begin to feel your eyes just straining a little as you stare at that spot there....while I talk to you....really aware of that spot there....and of how an interesting thing is beginning to happen to one of your arms....floating there....just above your legs...while you try to concentrate on looking at that spot....because everyone knows how easy it is, to learn something when you're comfortable.....and sooner or later everyone has the experience of learning something new when they're relaxed, so go ahead and allow that comfortable feeling to continue with the recognition that after a while you also can notice that your eyes naturally begin to get tired of staring at that spot, and it becomes difficult to keep holding them there, or even to keep them open.

And it really would be much easier....more comfortable to close them...and you might do that as staring at that blurry spot seems to be too much effort to bother making any more...but as you let them very slowly begin to close now....you can also notice, as they slowly close....a light floating feeling in one hand...or the other....or both....so that as eyelids feel heavy...and you continue to let them go down....an arm floats up a bit...and then a bit more....floating away from your leg....because as it feels lighter...the eyes may seem to feel heavier....but as your heavy eyes continue to close...your light floating arm moves upwards a bit more....as it feels even lighter than before....and you can feel it lifts upwards....drifts upwards...almost by itself at times....more and more......as you continue bit by bit....to close those heavy eyes...and your light lifting arm....floating up as you drift down with your eyes....arm lifting upwards at times...and then back down perhaps.....and then back upward again....an automatic movement upwards...one small step at a time...upward and then upward a bit more....like being pulled upward with a soft string....light as a feather...and it may be difficult to tell just how much that arm and hand have drifted up....to tell exactly what position they are in....and it may be difficult to tell when that slow effortless movement occurs more and more rapidly, as it drifts up lighter and lighter...higher and higher....that's right (pause for upward movement) ...and that arm and hand could continue to drift higher and get lighter and lighter.....but after a while you may begin to notice now....that as you allow your eyes to close comfortably now...and your mind to relax...that relaxed heaviness spreads ...and that arm begins to feel heavier too....as it begins to move back down.

And as you pay close attention to it...you may begin to notice how it feels now....how tired and heavy it is....as your unconscious mind reminds your mind....to pay more and more attention to how good it feels to go back down.

And that arm moves down now.....as that heaviness increases....because it would be so comfortable...just to allow that heavy arm to drift all the way down now....as you drift sown into a comfortable relaxation....eyes closed....arms relaxed....that's right...and drifting down with it....down into a deep, deep trance....as your arm relaxes and the mind relaxes as well....and you drift deeper and deeper as I continue to talk...eyes closed now....and your arms and hands feel so comfortable....your entire body comfortable....comfortable and relaxed..."

(Go to either a deepener, direct suggestions or a metaphor)

Deepeners – to be used after an induction

The Garden Script

"As you go deeper now..... your subconscious mind becomes open.... More accessible and receptive to new learning's.... To changing old beliefs.......as you relax so comfortably there.... Just listening to the sound of my voice.....here.....so calm....and a feeling of peace and tranquillity allows you to relax more and more......with each easy breath.....with each gentle beat of your heart. As I count down from ten to one......you can just let go and you can go deeper now......with each count.......using each number to let go of stress and tension..... to go deeper now.

Ten......As you allow each muscle and nerve in your body to relax......letting go......becoming calm......you feel peaceful.....comfortable now.

Nine......Relax your mind and your body together.......and if you lose track of the sequence of the numbers..... then that's fine......just let go now......as.....

Eight....... You start to sense a gentle connection between your mind and your body......and an inner wisdom.

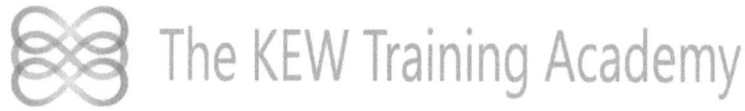

Seven.......Go deeper now......and as you breathe out........ *(Start to pace the persons breathing.)* ....start to breathe out any tension.......breathing out anxiety now.

Six.....letting any fear......anger or stress flow away from your body....with every outward breath.......letting go now......slowly......comfortably.....calmly.

Five.......And now with each outward breath......I want you to start saying a word to yourself......without moving your mouth or your tongue......your breathing not changing......your throat perfectly still......on each outward breath......say the word inwardly to yourself.....**calm**......(pace with outward breath.....and repeat)......*calm*...

Four......without thinking what it means.....without analysing the word.....just moving the sound inwards now ..... so that it seems to come from an inner wisdom....

(match breathing)

.....calm.....

Three.......*Gently now......easily......calmly.....calm......letting go.......and whenever your mind strays from that sound.......and it will stray away......then just acknowledge that fact and gently bring it back......repeating to yourself the word......***calm....**

(matching breathing)

Two...... Continuing now to relax.......and to let go....gently drifting down......into peace and harmony of body......mind.......and spirit......

One.....And as you continue to drift deeper still......you begin to see.....sense or imagine yourself in a beautiful garden......the sun is shining......gently warming your skin......comfortable....relaxed ...You look across the garden as it sweeps away to an ornamental pond......with a fountain playing......the water droplets sparkling......glistening......in the soft diffused light that filters down through the leaves and branches of the ancient trees that surround this magical garden....shielding and sheltering this beautiful place. The grass is soft.....springy beneath your feet.....and as you walk......you pass flower beds cut into the lawn....filled with the most beautiful flowers and plants......so many varieties and colours.....and you can be aware of the fragrance of the flowers carried to you on a soft breeze that drifts across the garden....rustling the leaves......causing the heads of the flowers to sway gently......the subtle sounds of nature all around you.....birds singing.....the soft sound of insects and the splash of cascading water.....each sound......each sensation......relaxing you even more......comforting you as you drift deeper......and every step becomes heavier.

You soon find yourself in a small clearing.....the sun warming you and relaxing you more and more now......as you sit.....resting your back against a large and ancient tree.... The bark of the tree is so soft and comfortable.....and you sense that many people have rested here as you are resting now.......and although you are alone......you feel safe here.....peaceful......comfortable.....the word **calm**....comforts you more and more as your mind drifts and fades."

Hypnotherapy Practitioner Course - Professional Accredited Hypnotherapy Training

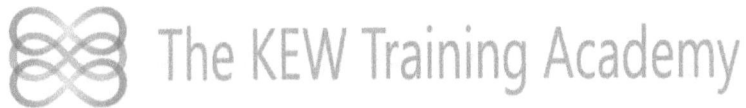
My Best Friend Script – Deepener

This deepener is a variation of Milton Erickson's "My Friend John" method. It works well for resistant subjects, as most people like to help others or show them what to do; consequently the subject, in showing his best friend how to go into trance, goes into trance himself (or herself).

"See that chair over there? I'd like you to imagine that your best friend is sitting there, wanting to be hypnotized, and that you're the one who is going to show him how to do it. So form an awareness of how your friend looks, whilst sitting there. Give the instructions to your friend after me (in your mind, if you wish)."

"Tell your best friend to close his eyes. Tell him to relax the tiny muscles around the eyes. Are they relaxed? Good, now tell him to relax all of the facial muscles and very slowly, very gradually, talk him through relaxing the rest of his body, working down from the head to the toes and the shoulders to the fingertips."

Give a long pause to allow your subject to carry out this instruction, intercepted with "that's right" "good", "relax", very softly. Watch your subject for muscle relaxation and change of skin colour.

"Now tell your best friend to breathe slowly, and deeply, in and out, deeper and deeper. Now tell him that in a moment one of his hands will begin to feel light and floaty. He might begin to wonder whether it will be the right hand or the left hand. Tell him that those fingers are lifting ever so slowly, ever so gently, off his lap (or wherever the hand is resting), and it is beginning to float all the way up."

This is an excellent tester to see how your subject is responding. By now his own hand should begin to lift, and when you observe the signs of this, encourage the movement by saying "lighter and lighter".

"And when his hand touches his face you will go into a very deep trance. You will hear everything that I say but you will feel so comfortably relaxed that you just want to sink deeper and deeper down into that wonderful feeling."

(If by chance the hand does not move at all, deepen the trance further by asking him to take his friend down a very steep staircase. Be sure first though that he is not afraid of heights.)

The Minds Eye – Deepener

An extremely effective technique that can be utilised to "dampen down" the continual internal self talk, allowing for deeper trance experience:

"In the same way that you have eyes that see the world around you, you also have an inner eye that we call "the minds eye"....and it can see images and process thoughts even as you relax so deeply....and the minds eye has an eyelid and, like your physical eye, that eyelid can close down....as it too becomes heavy and tired....wanting to close....and it can begin to close....and, as it slowly drops, it shuts out stray thoughts....stray images, and can leave your mind perfectly clear...it experiences whatever you would choose...and its closing

Hypnotherapy Practitioner Course - Professional Accredited Hypnotherapy Training

now...closing more and more....and your mind grows quiet and at peace...and now it closes completely...closing out all stray thoughts or images that you don't want to interfere with how relaxed you are...."

Creating a Brilliant Future Technique

This very powerful technique can be used to help clients with any kind of goal or outcome that they want to achieve. For example, weight loss, stopping smoking, overcoming fears, phobias, passing a driving test or exam, even healing.

1. Create an image of what your life will be like at some point in the future when you have achieved your goal/outcome.

2. Mark 2 pieces of paper on the floor – one that represents today and one for a time in the future when you will have achieved your outcome. The distance (time) between the two spots should be what feels right. Stand on the future spot and imagine what it is like having achieved your goal. Imagine you have a remote control like the one you use for your television. Use it to intensify the qualities of your internal imagery and sound. Turn up the brightness, increase the colour, improve the contrast, make it bigger and bring it closer. Turn up the volume and listen to the sounds. Have the sound tuned so that there is no interference. Step into the picture and notice the feelings of satisfaction and achievement. Enjoy the moment and anchor this state. (Set an Anchor – kinaesthetic, auditory – visual, Anchoring technique is explained later in the course)

3. Lay the cards at equal intervals between where you are standing now (future) and the spot representing "today".

4. Stand at a spot just beyond the "future" spot and look back at "today" Fire the anchor you set earlier, how does it feel, having achieved your outcome(s)? From this position what have you got to say to the you of today? Have you any tips or advice?

5. Move to the Identity card, ask yourself how you have changed, now that you have achieved your outcomes. What is different about you? What role are you now playing that you were not playing before?

6. Move to the Values & Beliefs card. What values have you changed, if any, and how have your beliefs changed in order to achieve success?

7. Move to the Capability spot. How have your capabilities changed? What did you learn along the way? Hypnotherapy Centre of Excellence - Hypnotherapy Practitioner Course www.hypnotherapy-trainingcourses.com

8. Move to the Behaviour card. What did you do along the way? What are you doing differently now?

9. Move on to the Environment card. What impact has achieving your outcome(s) had on those around you? Is your environment still the same or has it changed at all? If so, how?

Hypnotherapy Practitioner Course - Professional Accredited Hypnotherapy Training

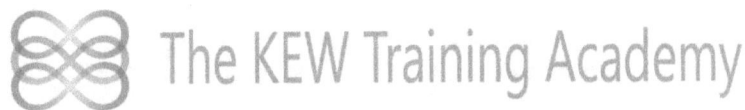
10. Revisit the cards in any order you wish if you feel that there is still work to do. You will know when you have true alignment as you will have a burning desire to make your first move towards achieving your goal.

This exercise can be done mentally after a short induction and deepener. Spacing the cards out on the floor is another way of doing the technique and can also be a very powerful way of (programming in) the changes you want to make and can sometimes give you a better concept of time that it will take.

Stress Management

Client Session for Stress Relief/ Management – Steps to Take

1. Consultation Building Rapport: Where/ when do you feel stressed? Where/when do you feel relaxed? "Where would you go to your own special place of relaxation"

2. What makes that place/experience relaxing? (Get clients own words and phrases – write them down to use in the session later)

3. Any Induction Script: Ticking clock, beautiful day, Fixation Script

4. Deepener: Garden, My Best Friend, Staircase – "each step takes you ten times deeper into relaxation"

5. Deepener – Dial "Turn up the feelings of relaxation to the very highest that they will go"

6. Stress relief script

7. Post Hypnotic Suggestions

8. Bring back out of trance state – counting back 1...2...3...

Stress Test

Please answer yes or no to the following questions. Please answer yes, even if only part of the question applies to you. Take your time, but please be totally honest with your answers.

Q1 I find that I don't have time for many interests / hobbies outside of work

Q2 I feel that there are just not enough hours in the day to do all of the things that I must do

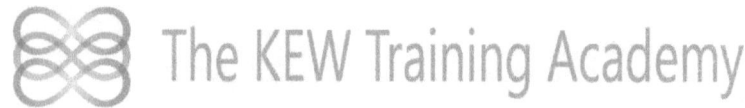

Q3 I find I have a greater dependency on alcohol, caffeine, nicotine or drugs (whether prescription or not)

Q4 At times I can have an extreme reluctance to go to work

Q5 I try to fit more and more tasks into less and less time, resulting in me not allowing time for any unforeseen problems that may arise

Q6 I feel that there are too many deadlines in my work / life that are difficult to meet

Q7 Lately my self-confidence / self-esteem is low

Q8 I can frequently have a vaguely guilty feeling if I relax and do nothing, even for short periods of time

Q9 I find myself thinking about problems to do with my personal / business / professional life, even when I am supposed to be engaged in recreational pursuits

Q10 I can have a feeling of intense fatigue, even when I wake after sleep

Q11 At times I am unable to perform work or tasks as well as I used to , or I feel my judgement is clouded / not as good as it was

Q12 I have a tendency to eat, talk, move and walk quickly

Q13 My appetite has altered, either to a desire to go on a binge, especially on sweet, sugary foods, or I have suffered a loss of appetite

Q14 I find myself becoming irritated / angry if the car or traffic in front of me seems to me to be going too slowly / Queuing makes me angry.

Q15 I can feel anger and resentment at nothing in particular a feeling that something is missing, but I don't know what

Q16 I'm aware that I try to get other people to hurry up / get on with it

Q17 At times I feel depressed, tearful, irritable, all- over tension, short tempered, unusual clumsiness, concentration / memory is impaired, excessive perspiration

Q18 I find that if I have to do repetitive tasks, I become impatient

Q19 I can seem to be listening to other people's conversation, even though I am in fact preoccupied with my own thoughts

Q20 My health is deteriorating, I am unwell quite often

Q21 I find myself grinding my teeth, especially if I am stressed or feeling impatient

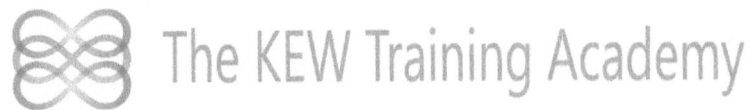

Q22 I seem to have an increase in aches and pains, especially in the neck, head, jaw, lower back, shoulders, and chest.

Score 1 for Yes **and 0 for No**

Reading the Results

4 points or less - No worries here.

5-13 points - You are prone to stress and may suffer from stress related illnesses.

14 points or more - You may need to think about getting some help managing these high levels of stress in your life.

The Weight of a Burden

A lecturer, when explaining stress management to an audience, raised a glass of water and asked, "How heavy is this glass of water?"Answers called out ranged from 20g to 500g.The lecturer replied, "The absolute weight doesn't matter. It depends on how long you try to hold it. If I hold it for a minute, that's not a problem.If I hold it for an hour, I'll have an ache in my right arm. If I hold it for a day, you'll have to call an ambulance. In each case, it's the same weight, but the longer I hold it, the heavier it becomes."

He continued, "And that's the way it is with stress management. If we carry our burdens all the time, sooner or later, as the burden becomes increasingly heavy, we won't be able to carry on. As with the glass of water, you have to put it down for a while and rest before holding it again. When we're refreshed, we can carry on with the burden."

Before you return home tonight, put the burden of work down. Don't carry it home. You can pick it up tomorrow. Whatever burdens you're carrying now, let them down for a moment if you can." So, why not take a while to just simply RELAX. Put down anything that may be a burden to you right now. Don't pick it up again until after you've rested a while. Life is short. Enjoy it!

Wash Away Stress Script - Sandcastles

As you begin to really enjoy this wonderful, relaxing feeling - I wonder if you'd like to discover a way of washing away all the stress and tension that you've been experiencing over the last few weeks and months?

I want you to imagine yourself on a lovely secluded beach - and it's a warm summer's day - the sun is shining down on you and it makes you feel good - it helps you to feel even more relaxed - and you can hear the sound of the waves and perhaps the call of a seabird far away.

And as you visualize this scene - perhaps you can find a particular memory that springs to mind - from your childhood days of a trip or a holiday to the seaside?

Did you ever build sandcastles as a child? If so, perhaps you can remember sitting down on the soft warm sand with a bucket and spade, filling the bucket with golden sand and patting it down when the sand piled over the top? Then turning it upside down and hitting the underside of the bucket with your spade to release the mould of sand.

You could build castle after castle - and when you were finished - scrape a moat in the sand around the castles and fill it with sea water - brought from the sea in your bucket - and perhaps even a makeshift flag to decorate your castle.

Well, we're going to do this now - so I want you to imagine yourself with a bucket and spade on this lovely beach - make this image real - be aware of the smell of the fresh salt sea air - the warmth of the sun on your skin - the feel of the soft golden sand beneath your bare feet - the sound of the waves as they gently splash - and perhaps even a gentle breeze on your skin and your hair.

Notice the sunlight glistening here and there on the sea - like millions of diamonds sparkling alluringly - palm trees with single, un-branching trunks topped with a tuft of fan-like or feather-like leaves - and whatever else comes into your mind - right now. And all those stresses and worries and cares can go into the bucket - with the sand - just pile it all in - maybe there are problems at work/school/home? Put those problems into the bucket - you really don't need them here.

Or maybe you have worries about a particular relationship in your life? If so - Put those worries into the bucket - and know that whatever will be - will be. And when one door closes another one invariably opens.

Perhaps you've been concerned about money or other material issues? In this peaceful place that you have created - materialistic issues just aren't important to you so pile them all into the bucket.

And when the bucket is full - turn it over and make your first sandcastle - here in hypnosis - hitting all your cares and worries and problems - together with the sand - to make your first mound.

When the bucket is empty you can consider any other problems that you may have in your life. If there are problems with family, other relatives, friends or anyone else that you know - put those problems into the bucket. You really don't need to be stressed any more.

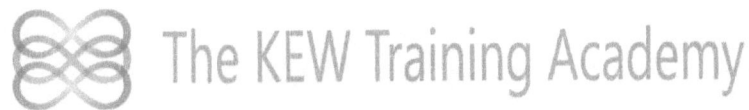

I'm going to be quiet for a few moments and I want you to go through any negative influences in your life and spade them all - every one of them - into the bucket - and when the bucket is full - make another mound to become part of your sandcastle.

And when you're finished - I want you to imagine standing up and taking a really good look at what you have created. All these problems seem so insignificant compared to the vast beach and sea and the sky. You really don't need to feel stressed any more - in any way.

Now - imagine yourself as a bird - flying up in the sky - looking down on the sandcastles that you've built and noticing how much smaller they now are.

As you look down at this birds eye view - a huge wave suddenly washes over the sand - and your sandcastle is gone - taking away all your worries and cares - and the sea becomes calm once again. Hear the sound of those now gentle waves - splashing easily and lazily - back and forth - to and fro - so soothing - so calming - so relaxing - and you take into yourself this soothing - calming - relaxing feeling.

An amazing thing happens to you - you find all those problems that were once on your mind are no longer there. They seem smaller - less significant - less bothersome - and suddenly you begin to see this in proportion - as they really are.

Experience this feeling of calmness now - enjoy it - memorize it - and in a moment or two when I count you up out of hypnosis – you can bring back with you those wonderful feelings and keep them with you - remembering them whenever you need to - whenever you want to.

I'm going to count up from one to five and at the count of five you will be fully alert and refreshed - you will have wonderful feelings flowing through your body - calm and peaceful thoughts flowing through your mind - and these lovely calm and peaceful thoughts and feelings are going to remain and stay with you.

So - when you're ready - one - two - three - coming slowly back - four - eyelids beginning to flutter and five - eyes open - wide awake - refreshed and alert - mind and body returning to normality.

Blow Away Stress Script

(Begin with your favourite induction and deepener.)

You are now deeply relaxed and the suggestions that you hear will have a permanent and immediate effect on your subconscious mind - you will hear every word that I speak - even though you may find your mind wandering away at times - because right now - nothing else matters - nothing - except for this wonderful feeling of relaxation that you're experiencing.

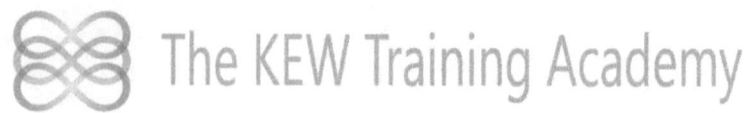

At this moment is as though you haven't a care in the world - nobody wants anything - nobody needs anything - there is absolutely nothing at all for you to do except relax and let go - and just enjoy these wonderful feelings that are being generated within you - now.

And I would like you to compare this feeling of complete relaxation to the unnecessary, unwanted and useless feelings that you've been experiencing lately - those feelings of being stressed out and anxious.

I'm sure that you already know how you prefer to feel - but in your normal, everyday life experiences you seemed to get wound up and irritated at the slightest thing - staying calm in a difficult situation didn't seem to come naturally to you.

This could have been because worries - about possibly mundane things - appeared to be piling up - and up - rather like placing one heavy book on another - until the whole pile of books became so heavy that you just could not lift them - and even thinking about lifting those books - or worrying about which one to remove first - just made the whole situation worse.

I would like you to think of each of those books as a worry - or a problem that has been in your life. Each of those books has a title - perhaps there is one called 'Work (or School) Worries - another called Colleagues (or Friends) - perhaps there is a Financial Book - I'm sure you know all the things that have been contributing to the stress that you've been experiencing - so go over this in your mind - whilst I'm quiet for a few moments.

(Pause)

Let me know by nodding your head when you've identified all the stress factors in your life. (Wait for signal) That's good - now I want you to leave those books on a table and in your imagination - come outside to a beautiful garden.

And it's a lovely warm day - the sun is shining and the sky is a perfect shade of blue - not a cloud in sight. You can have anything you like in your garden - your favourite flowers, a cascading waterfall and a beautiful rustic arch that is covered with fragrant flowers of blue and pink and purple. Over there are two very strong trees and if you look carefully you will see the hammock that is strung between them.

A few steps lead up to the hammock so you climb inside - making yourself even more comfortable - even more relaxed and detached - detached and relaxed.

And ever so gently you swing from side to side - side to side - by a baby in a rocking cradle - lulling gently to sleep - and it's such a comfortable feeling - and so perfect to be here right now that you want to hold this feeling to you - forever.

And you can - you really can feel wonderful - and so relaxed and comfortable.

In your hammock you notice something that you hadn't seen before - it is a brightly coloured container with a screw lid - just small enough to fit in your hand as it is cylindrical in shape. You unscrew the lid and are delighted to find that it's a bubble blower - the type you probably played with when you were a small child. The container is full of rainbow coloured liquid and you dip the stick with the rounded bit into the liquid and blow your first bubble. As you watch the bubble dancing in the light summer breeze - a thought suddenly occurs to you that each bubble could represent one of the issues that had been causing you to feel stressed.

Do you remember the titles of those books? Okay - so one by one you dip the wand into the container and think of a title - perhaps Work or School pressures - blow the bubble now - gently at first as the bubble begins to form - and then blow it away - just blow it away - that's right - blow your worries about work or school away. The have no right to bother you whilst you are relaxed and comfortable.

And as soon as you blow that bubble away - all worries about work or school just disappear - and you realize that you don't need to be stressed - you can be calm - relaxed - and comfortable - that's right - so wonderfully calm and relaxed and comfortable.

Think of another title now - perhaps worries about family or friends or colleagues - and just blow your bubble - gently at first as the bubble begins to form - then blow it out of your life - just blow it away - it has no right to make you feel stressed - you now realize that there are far better ways of thinking and feeling - and stress isn't one of them - you much prefer to feel calm, relaxed and comfortable.

Repeat this process with any other worries that have been making you stressed - blow each one of them out of your life - I will be quiet for a few moments - and when you're sure they're are gone, nod your head as a signal to me.

(Wait for signal).

That's good. Now your body and mind know how to relax - and blow those stressful thoughts or feelings out of your life - and you can imagine doing this if every any of those old worries - or new ones - try to bother you in the future - just blow them away - you don't want them - you don't need them and you certainly won't have them - so you blow them out of your life.

And as you do - you immediately feel so much calmer, so much more relaxed and so much more comfortable too.

And because of your new found ability to relax - you find yourself becoming so much more confident in all areas of your life. And these suggestions are firmly embedded in your subconscious mind and grow stronger and stronger day by day. They grow stronger by the day, stronger by the hour, stronger by the minute. In a moment I'm going to count the numbers from one to five and at the count of five you will be wide awake, feeling already wonderfully invigorated - and ready to allow these suggestions - to work for you. One, two, three, coming slowly back - four - eyelids beginning to flutter and five - eyes open - wide awake - mind and body returning to normality.

Stress Relief with Hypnosis

Imagine you're sat in a comfortable place, watching a lit candle in front of you on a table.

I want you to focus your eyes on the flame of the candle, just watch it flicker and dance, lose yourself in its warmth that's good keep focused on the flame jumping and dancing.

As you watch the flame I want you to notice your breathing and how your abdomen rises as you breath in the calming warmth of the candle flame, now take three, long, deep breaths for me, taking in with each deep, slow breath, the relaxing warm feeling of the candle flame as you do so, and just let your eyes close now.

As you sit here becoming more relaxed focus on my voice now, and allow yourself to become more and more relaxed; and allow yourself to relax deeper knowing that you are fully aware of all the sounds in the room, but these sounds just help you to go deeper still because should you need to become fully awake during this, or any hypnotic state, all you need to do is count up from one to five and you will be fully awake fully awake; fully alert and able to deal with whatever situation awaits you.

So now as you lay here, I want you to imagine you're laid on a beach, or in a garden, and it is a lovely clear warm day with a bright sun in the sky. You can feel that soothing warmth in the muscles on the top of your head. The warmth is so soothing, it relaxes all the muscles of the scalp, feel them loosen and relax, that's good, now let that relaxation and warmth flow down into the muscles of your face, around the eyes, into the cheeks and the jaw, that's right just let your jaw loosen and allow a gap to form between your top and bottom teeth, and let your tongue drop from the roof of your mouth that's good, so now your whole head and face are wonderfully relaxed.

I want you to allow this wonderful relaxing warm feeling to flow down into your neck and shoulders from the face, that's good feel the muscles of the neck and those long muscles of the shoulders loosen and relax, that's right just let the shoulders sag and loosen more and more, now allow this wonderful feeling to flow down into your arms loosening and relaxing both arms, those long bicep muscles lengthen and expand and feel relaxed and heavy. now down into the fingers of both hands this feeling of relaxation spreads. You may feel tingling or lightness in one or both hands as you relax even deeper and that is fine if you do.

You're doing wonderfully now, and I want you to allow the relaxing warmth to flow into your chest relaxing all the muscles of the chest feel them loosen now and this feeling this warm lovely feeling flows into your abdomen releasing all the tension from your stomach

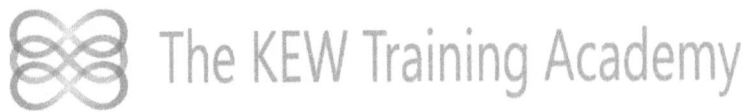

muscles, and you can notice now the softness of the chair as you allow your spine to be loose just like a piece of rope and allow your body to relax further and sink into the chair.

Your relaxation is deeper than ever now, and you feel wonderful as you allow the warm feeling to flow into your legs through your pelvic area, allow the long muscles of the thigh to relax and expand becoming loose, now the feeling flows through the knees into the calves and ankles, down to your feet and toes. Your whole body is totally relaxed and at ease and you can return to this state at any time in the future and it feels wonderful to know this.

I want you to imagine you're at the top of a wonderful staircase it is a well lit beautiful stair case with ten steps leading down, in a moment we are going to walk down these stairs one at a time and as I count you down each step you will go deeper into hypnosis, OK here we go take the first step down now 10 deeper and deeper, more and more relaxed 9 that's good deeper and deeper now 8 more relaxed deeper 7 6 deeper more relaxed more relaxed and deeper still 5 deeper with each step now 4 more relaxed 3 deeper 2 totally at ease and peace 1 that's excellent.

In front of you is a door I want you to walk through it and as you do, there is a shield in front of the door, it is an invisible force field which will not allow negative feelings or bad habits through, they will be left behind and will not bother you again, that's good step through into a lovely calm place, this is your tranquil place where you can come at anytime, it can be a room or a beach or anywhere you feel totally at ease, totally relaxed.

You are now deeply relaxed and ready to accept the suggestions I give, I want you to now remember a time when you were uptight and tense but I want you to see it as a bystander, see the worried look on the face of this other person, a person who looks like you but is not you, see the worry on his brow the tension in his eyes, the way he arches as the tension tightens his stomach muscles notice how he clenches his facial muscles with the strain.

You can see and acknowledge and feel this persons tensions because they are your tensions, but unlike in past times now you can recognize these signs and you can deal with them. As you see this person stood beside you now, know the signs you see in him are in you, see the look on his face and know it on your own face and as we learn today and here after that should your signs of tension start to appear, you can deal with them.

All you need to do is to make a fist and as you make the fist, feel the tension and nervousness and all the negative energy flow from your brow, your stomach and every area of your body to your fist, and as the energy flows to your fist, the fist tightens, tighter and tighter until all the negative feelings thoughts and energy are all in your hand.

Now you can open your fist and see this negative energy flow away it blows away in the wind like grains of sand insignificant small and unable to bother you again.

Any time from now on when you see the tensions building up you feel wonderful knowing that you can close your eyes, take 5 deep breaths, make a fist with either hand, and pull all

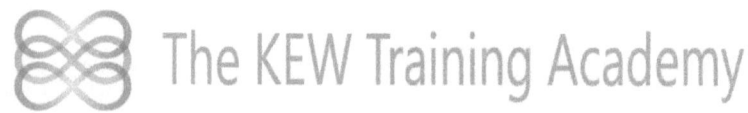
the tension into a fist, acknowledge the fist of tension and its cause, and then release the fist and the tension for ever, feeling better and better as day by day you find less and less things make you tense, and you feel happier and more relaxed as each day goes by.

Now in a moment I am going to count from 1 to 10 and as I count with each number, you will come nearer and near to full normal awaked ness, your whole body will feel invigorated alive and full of energy to take on the day. OK here we go 1 feeling more awake now 2 more alert 3 full of energy, 4 more and more awake 5, nearer and nearer to full awakeness 6 feeling wonderful 7 more and more awake 8 your whole body is awake lively and feeling marvellous 9 right at the top now, fully awake whole body totally awake and alive 10 eyes open wide awake feeling totally wonderful.

Overcoming Fears & Phobias

What is Fear?

Fear is a normal part of your everyday life; it prevents you from coming to harm and getting hurt. When a fear starts to have a negative impact on your everyday life and prevents you from doing everyday things then it becomes a phobia.

For example, you may have a fear of walking through the park when its dark at night time, or crossing a busy road and this may be perfectly normal, but when your fear starts to become of walking through the park even when its daytime and safe and there are other people around, it starts to have an impact in your life then it becomes a phobia.

We are not born with fear, we pick them up throughout life. Phobias are mainly picked up from those around us, which is known as a learnt fear, or from experiences that we have.

Just as we can learn to have a phobia, we can also "un-learn" using hypnotherapy to re-programme the mind and change the meaning and association that we give to experiences.

A great way of getting an insight into a client's mind, someone that we may never have met before is to ask them

"If I was to be you for the day and was to have your phobia, what would I have to experience?"

"How would you teach me to have your phobia, what would I have to picture in my mind, what sounds would I have to hear, what feelings would I have to experience? Any tastes or smells associated to having your phobia?"

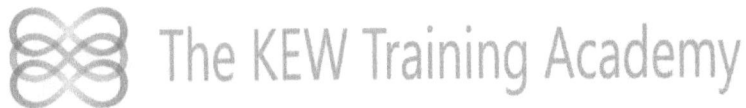

A Brief Explanation of Fears & Phobias A Fear:

This is an emotional response to a threat. It is a basic survival mechanism occurring in response to a specific stimulus, such as pain or the threat of danger. Fear should not be confused with anxiety as this usually occurs without any external threat.

A Phobia:

This is an intense reaction or irrational reaction to something or some situation. The sufferer will; experience feelings that appear to be completely out of their control. The sufferer will actively ensure that they never allow themselves to be in any situation that could cause phobic reaction. Specific phobias can be categorised and I have listed four:

- **Animal Phobias:** Spiders, Snakes, Dogs, Cats etc.

- **Natural Environment:** Heights, Fire, Water, Thunderstorms and the dark.

- **Blood / Injury /Needles:** Injections, the sight of blood, dentistry, surgical operations, or other invasive medical procedures.

- **Situational:** Flying, lifts, driving, tunnels, bridges, enclosed spaces (Claustrophobia), or being sick.

Top 10 Common Phobias

1. **Arachnophobia:** The fear of spiders. This phobia tends to affect women more than men.

2. **Ophidiophobia:** The fear of snakes. Often attributed to evolutionary causes, personal experiences, or cultural influences.

3. **Acrophobia:** The fear of heights. This fear can lead to anxiety attacks and avoidance of high places.

4. **Agoraphobia:** The fear of situations in which escape is difficult. This may include crowded areas, open spaces, or situations that are likely to trigger a panic attack. People will begin avoiding these trigger events, sometimes to the point that they cease leaving their home. Approximately one third of people with panic disorder develop agoraphobia.

5. **Cynophobia:** The fear of dogs. This phobia is often associated with specific personal experiences, such as being bitten by a dog during childhood.

6. **Astraphobia:** The fear of thunder and lightning. Also known as Brontophobia, Tonitrophobia, or Ceraunophobia.

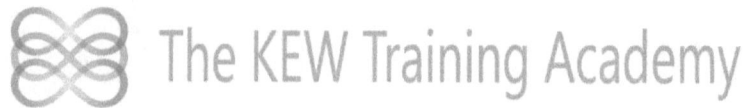
7. **Trypanophobia:** The fear of injections. Like many phobias, this fear often goes untreated because people avoid the triggering object and situation.

8. **Social Phobias:** The fear of social situations. In many cases, these phobias can become so severe that people avoid events, places, and people that are likely to trigger an anxiety attack.

9. **Pteromerhanophobia:** The fear of flying. Often treated using exposure therapy, in which the client is gradually and   progressively introduced to flying.

10. **The fear of germs or dirt:** May be related to obsessive-compulsive disorder.

The Fast Phobia Cure Technique

a. Get as much information as possible from the client about their Phobia, where and when they usually have the phobia. Ask them "If I had to be you for the day and you had to teach me how to have your phobia, what would I have to experience?" What would I have to see, hear and feel? Elicit all the sub modalities in the pre-talk before beginning the technique.

b. Ask them on a scale of 1 to 10 how severe their phobia is at present

c. Get the client to draw a picture of the phobia as it is in their mind at the moment, very often a picture can tell a thousand words and give a good insight into what the client is picturing in their mind. You can ask the client to draw another picture of the phobia once the technique has been completed to see if there are any changes.

d. It is then useful to have the client draw up a list of all the advantages and disadvantages of holding on to this phobia. This helps to show the client that there are more disadvantages and how holding on to this phobia is affecting their life.

e. Begin the technique with a relaxation script by asking your client to close their eyes, focus on their breathing and relax. Ask your client to recall a time when they felt really relaxed and calm and ask them to relive those calm relaxing feelings. The "Wash Away Stress Sandcastle Script" can also be used here to help get your client into a relaxed state of mind.

f. Have you client walk into an"imaginary movie theatre" in their mind and sit down somewhere comfortable and relaxing.

g. Have them float up out of their body and gently settle in a comfortable seat in the balcony, so they can watch themselves watching the screen.

h. Have them put the very beginning of their Phobia on the screen in the form of a movie in full colour. At all times remind them that they are just observing and that

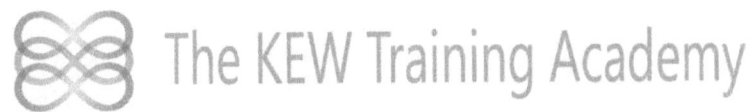
there are no feelings involved. Have them run the movie of their phobia all the way to end, as they remain in the balcony watching sitting in the front row watching themselves on the screen. (Completely detached from any feelings)

i.   At the end of the movie, freeze the frame into a slide. Change the picture to black and white draining any colours, ask them to turn the sounds right down and to add some funny music that makes them laugh. Run the movie backwards at triple speed or faster, with the funny music playing, then have them fast forward the movie, then keep re-winding and fast forwarding the movie as fast as they can 3 times then have them freeze - frame the image when they get to the beginning of the movie.

j.   Then ask them to white out the entire screen letting go of any association to the situation in the movie. The client is still listening to the funny music at all times.

k.   Have your client leave the movie theatre feeling relaxed and calm leaving any associations to the phobia behind, reminding them that they are starting a new chapter and all of the things that they will now be able to do. Test for the phobic response by asking your client to imagine themselves in a situation that may in the past have brought on the phobic response. Have your client continue to listen to the funny music, reminding them that they no longer have any association to the phobia.

l.   End the technique by bringing your client back into the room by counting them back from 1 to 3 then asking them to open their eyes.

m.   Ask the client again on a scale of 1 to 10 how severe the phobia is now and if their association to it has now changed.

n.   Ask the client to now draw a picture of their phobia to see if there are any changes to the original drawing in step 3.

Abreactions/Cathartic Release

An abreaction is a strong association to a negative emotion or feeling connected to a perceived past event. They are rare but can be quite extreme and need to be dealt with in the appropriate way.

How to Take Control of an Abreaction

1. STAY CALM – You are the authority figure – so you must stay calm and remain in control of the situation so the client feels safe.

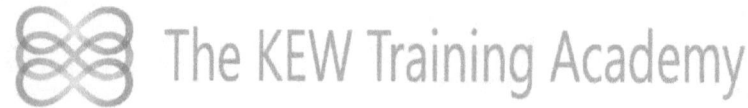
2. DO NOT TOUCH – Any touch at this stage can act as an anchor, if you were to give a client a hug and a rub of the back or shoulder this can create a physiological anchor that may be triggered at a later stage when the client's wife gives them a hug.

3. SAFE PLACE: Remind them that they can view or sense the events from a safe place (that you will have established in the pre-talk/consultation) so that they do not have to view or sense what is happening directly.

4. IF YOU FEEL CONFIDENT/HAVE EXPERIENCE: Gently guide the client through the emotional release. Offer encouragement such as: That's right; Moving through that now; You're doing really well etc. Only if you feel confident or have Hypnosis experience should you let the client move through the Abreaction. If you can allow this to happen, amazing healing can take place.

5. COUNT THEM OUT OF HYPNOSIS: Once it all feels complete and you have asked the client if it does and the session feels like it is at a close, then count them out of Hypnosis.

Self Hypnosis Techniques

Self Hypnosis is a great technique to teach clients as a way of managing stress and inducing relaxation.

Self Hypnosis can be used to help overcome any habit, and facilitate any behavioral change. Plus teaching a client self hypnosis techniques and telling them to use the techniques regularly will give the client responsibility for overcoming their problem and will help them gain control over their mind and getting to where they want to be.

Self Hypnosis is very powerful and is a great way of focussing on the outcome that you want to happen and creating new neurological pathways in the mind.

The Seven Step Self Hypnosis Process

1. Identify the problem or concern that you want to address and plan it on your template. You can copy the template to create as many as you wish.

2. Induce trance. Firstly find a quiet place to relax and lie down, somewhere where you will not be disturbed. You can use some relaxing music if it helps you to relax more easily, Stare at a spot on the ceiling until your eyes begin to feel strained and tired, then relax them down, close them and take 3 deep breaths in. then just focus on your breathing and bring to mind the last time that you felt deeply relaxed, comfortable and imagine going right back there now, allowing those feelings of relaxation to flow through every part of your body. If you can't remember a time when you felt relaxed then imagine how it would feel in your ideal situation to be completely relaxed and at ease, allow those feelings to get stronger.

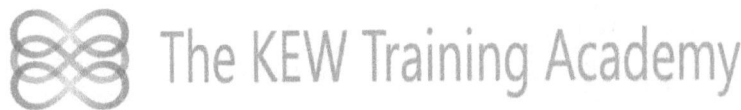
3. Now focus on what you will do as your solution – imaging how you will think, feel and act.

4. Visualize yourself carrying out the new behaviour. This is your mental rehearsal.

5. State positive affirmations that you can easily repeat to yourself to remind yourself about the changes that you are creating.

6. Now make your own posthypnotic suggestion with this easy formula: "From now on whenever I encounter (the problem), I am now doing (the new behaviour)"

7. Reorient yourself: open your eyes, stretch and take a deep breath. Done!

The KEW Training Academy

Self Hypnosis Template

Step 1. Problem or concern

____

____

____

___ ____

Step 2. Self Hypnosis Induction: Take a deep breath and focus your attention on a spot on the ceiling.

Step 3: Create the solution: how you want to respond differently – how you will think act and feel.

*New thinking:*____

____

____

*New feeling:*____

____

____

*New actions:*____

____

____

Step 4. Visualize yourself carrying out the solution in a situation that previously would have been challenging. This is your mental rehearsal.

____

____

____

Step 5. Your positive affirmations:

____

____

____

____

____

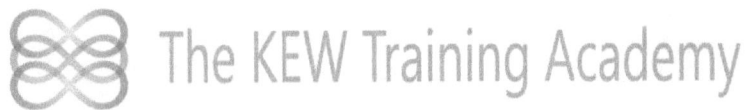
Step 6. Your posthypnotic suggestion: From now on whenever I encounter

_____

_____

I Will

_____

_____

_____

Step 7. Reorient yourself: Open your eyes, stretch, and take a deep breath

Ideomotor Response (I.M.R)

There are many occasions in therapy where it is necessary to ask the client questions and to receive answers. It is a widely held belief that sometimes asking the client to speak during hypnosis can interfere with the depth of the trance.

So in order to avoid this, the client is asked to communicate via finger movements to signal yes or no. This technique is known as Ideomotor signalling /response.

Calm Switch Technique

This technique can be taught to a client to help them to stay calm and relaxed in any situation. It is always a good idea to teach your client techniques that they can take away and use themselves as this promotes self responsibility and enables the client to learn to manage their own feelings.

Tell client to close their eyes or use an Induction.

Say ... Remember a time when you felt calm, really, really calm. Fully return to it now...see what you saw, hear what you heard and feel how good it felt... If you cannot remember a time, imagine how good it would feel If you were very confident and had all the power and strength and self-belief you could ever need.

1.   As you keep going through this memory...make the colours richer and bolder...the sounds louder and clearer and the feelings stronger.

2.   As you feel those calm relaxed feelings increase, squeeze the thumb and middle finger of right hand together.

3.   Now really squeeze the thumb and middle finger together and relive that good feeling.

4.   **Repeat steps one to five several times with different calm relaxing memories** until just squeezing your thumb and finger together brings back those good feelings. **(Alternatively, say)...**you will notice as you touch finger and thumb together that instantly those calm relaxed feelings return now.

Still holding finger and thumb together, think of a time or situation in which you used to feel stressed. Now imagine things going perfectly, going exactly as you want them to and feel how good that feels to be much calmer and in control of the situation.

5.   Still holding finger and thumb together, imagine a few challenging situations occurring and notice yourself handling them all easily and just in the way, you wanted. Notice how good that feels to be calm and in control.

6.   Each time you repeat this exercise it will become easier and easier to experience feelings of calm and relaxation 'at your fingertips'.

Weight Loss using Hypnotherapy

Different kinds of eaters Emotional Eaters

Emotional eaters are people who tend to eat food in response to their emotions such as stress, loneliness, upset, worry, frustration, boredom, lack of love in their life, punishment or they will even use food as a reward. This type of eater is also known as a comfort eater. They are trying to feed their emotions with food.

Conditioned Eaters

A conditioned eater tends to over eat food normally due to early childhood conditioning where the child was possibly made to feel guilty for leaving any leftover food on their plate at meal times. They may have been told that there "are starving people in other countries so they must eat the food" or the child may have been motivated to eat everything on their plate in order to get the dessert. So pleasure has been associated to eating all of the foods in front of them, and guilt to not eating the food.

Being rewarded as a child for "being good" with sweets or giving children sweets and junk food when they are upset conditions them so that later in life they still see these bad foods as a comfort and a connection to the love that they had as a child.

Subconscious Eaters

A subconscious eater tends to be totally unaware of the amount of food that they eat, for example they may be watching a film and without realising it they have eaten a whole giant bag of popcorn or a tub of ice cream. This type of eater is continuously snacking at work and

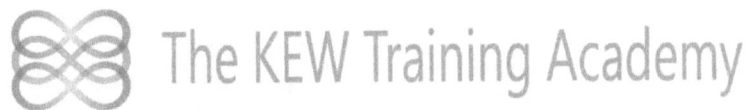

is not aware of how much they are actually eating throughout the day. A subconscious eater is an automatic eater and is not aware of their overeating habit.

SIMPLE UNNATURAL GLUCOSE, ADDITIVE REFINED, Pure White & Deadly – The Cocaine of the Food World.

Your body can't digest sugar – it transfers some of the sugar to the liver and muscles for "short term" energy use – **THE REST IS TRANSPORTED TO YOUR FAT CELLS!!!!**

"If you don't look after your body you'll have nowhere to live!"

1lb of fat = 3,500calories

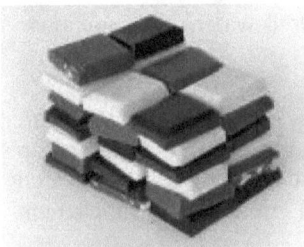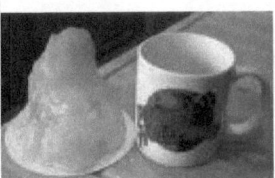

Consequences of eating Sugar Bitter sweet

Some of the dangers of consuming refined sugar are well known - tooth decay and obesity - but sugar can also suppress the immune system, and upset the body's mineral balance. It can reduce helpful high-density cholesterol (HDLs) and promote an elevation of harmful cholesterol (LDLs).

Sugar can cause hypoglycaemia, hormonal imbalance, varicose veins, food allergies, hypertension and depression. Sugar is also addictive; it can cause cravings for more food, particularly sweet food, leading to over-eating.

Sugar Addiction

Tips on how to kick the sugar habit

Some experts believe kicking sugar is harder than kicking cigarettes or even heroine!

Sugar is everywhere. It is advertised on television, at parties, in drinks, and hidden in many foods. So, to get the sugar out of your diet, where do you start? The tips below will get you started.

1. **Know all the sneaky names for sugar.** Read food labels and get rid of condiments, sauces, and dressings with sugar in them. Learn to make condiments and dressings without the sugar.

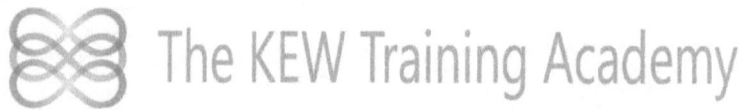
2. **Eat fruit.** Fruit is a great way to eat something sweet, and control calories. Just stay away from dried fruit or sweetened fruit.

3. **Avoid artificial sweeteners.** These are just a crutch. They keep you from learning to enjoy the natural sweetness of real food. There are also studies that show that they can make you crave sugar, not to mention the studies that show other dangerous health effects like cancer.

4. **Eliminate the white stuff.** White flour, white rice, and white potatoes. These have the same effect on blood sugar as sugar, and this will make sugar harder to kick. These foods keep you on the **insulin- low blood sugar cycle.**

5. **Avoid juice.** Even 100% juice is sugar water in disguise. Drink water, and if you must, only a splash of juice for flavour.

6. **Try stevia.** Stevia is an herb that is very sweet and has a slight liquorice flavour. While it is a stretch to make a whole dessert with stevia, it is great in coffee and on cereal. It may take some getting used to, but it is way better than loading your food with sugar or known toxic chemicals. Tip: Look for stevia in the dietary supplement section. It will not be with the sweeteners.

7. **Learn to use honey.** If you really need a sugar fix, eat some honey. Learn to cook with it. Learn how to drizzle it in thin steams. It is very high in sugar but, has other benefits that sugar does not and it is all natural. **Tip:** Buy honey local to your area. The local pollens the bees use to make the honey could help prevent some seasonal allergies.

8. **Limit alcohol.** Alcohol is made from sugar. It acts like sugar in the body. Especially when you first are trying to kick sugar stay away from any alcoholic beverages.

9. **Bring a low sugar dessert to share.** Temptations are everywhere. Show others how delicious a low sugar life style can be.

10. **Keep it out of the house.** Do not temp yourself with your child's pop tarts or your husband's ice cream. Tell your family what you are doing and then put your foot down. It is hard enough without sweets calling your name all day long.

11. **Eat sweet potatoes, red potatoes, and brown rice with meals.** These are the foods to replace the white foods with. Sweet potatoes make a yummy dessert with a little yogurt. Steam small red potatoes or some brown rice to eat with dinner. If time is an issue, cook these items ahead of time.

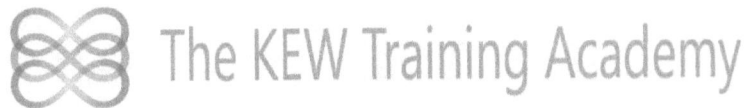
12. **If you must eat sweets, eat them after meals.** After meals sugar has less of an effect on blood sugar. You will be less likely to crash and crave more later.

Sugar can be kicked with Hypnotherapy and the cravings will lessen with time. The longer sugar is out of your diet the easier it gets.

"Everything you eat today will affect how you feel tomorrow"

Weight Loss Session Structure

- Weight Loss questionnaire

- Pre- Talk – start off with an outcome in mind, set some realistic compelling goals.

- To lose weight we need to burn off more calories than we consume.

- What exercise do you currently do? What exercise could you do?

- Find some activities that the client enjoys that they will stick to. Write them down, times, days that they will carry them out, with whom, when where?

- It takes 3,500 calories to burn off 1lbs of fat

- Weight Loss diagram – not on a diet, it's a new healthy way of eating.

- Explain the mind and how it works

- Make a list of their post hypnotic suggestions – in their own words to use later in the session.

- Dietary plan? Food swaps?

- Get Commitment from client – say hypnotherapy is extremely powerful and we have a very high success rate, are you definitely ready and committed to changing and moving forward with your life?

- Induction

- Deepener

- Therapy Script

- Post Hypnotic Suggestions

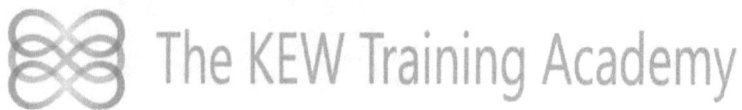
Exercise and Weight Loss

To lose one pound of fat, you must burn approximately 3500 calories **over and above what you already burn doing daily activities**. This obviously depends on your weight at the moment, and other factors which contribute towards your BMR, Basic Metabolic Rate which is the number of calories you burn are day at rest for example what your body needs to maintain normal functions like breathing, digestion, etc

Nutrition and calories

McDonald's double cheeseburger contains around 860 calories

To burn off the calories in just that *one* burger, the average 150- pound person would have to do moderate-intensity aerobics for well over an hour and a half!

Add on a shake and order of fries and you might as well cancel any plans you had for the half-a-day you'll need to spend at the gym to un-do that one meal!

Good nutrition is very important for fat loss, and focusing on health and health promoting foods is far more productive than focusing on fat loss and denial of favourite foods.

Make Exercise Fun

- Swimming pool

- Classes
  Sports: such as badminton, tennis, squash, anything you enjoy

- Gym circuit training

- Dancing

- Horse riding

- Rock climbing

- Table tennis

The list is exhaustive, identify activities you enjoy doing and integrate them into activity plan. Doing the activities you enjoy will help you to stay motivated, contribute towards a healthier life style.

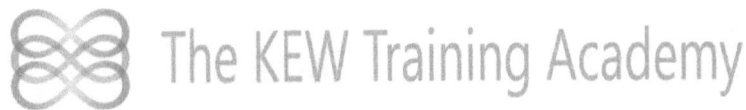
Goal Setting: Have a goal: e.g. sign up for a 5 km Fun Run. You can start losing weight **right now** by making a few simple changes. If you can burn around an extra 500 calories each day, you'll lose a pound a week. Try these ideas:

Instead of....

_____

Do this...

_____

Having an afternoon Coke

Drink a glass of water. (calories saved: 97)

Eating a bacon sandwich for breakfast

Eat some fruit and cereal (calories saved: 185)

Using your break to catch up on work or eat a snack

Go for a walk (calories burned: 100)

Wake up 5 minutes early

Get up 10 minutes early to some exercises, I.e. abdominal crunches (calories burned: 100)

Watching television after work

Do 10 minutes of yoga

So how does this goal setting technique work?

1. State your goal in the positive.

Think about what you want rather than what you don't want. If you still come up with something negative ask yourself "What do I want instead?" In the context of weight loss what do you want?

2. State it in simple terms.

If a five year old wouldn't understand it, it may be too complex - unlike some goal setting techniques your goal needs to be brief, simple and specific. I.e. how many pounds do you want to lose and when, what dress size would you like to fit in to, what size jeans?

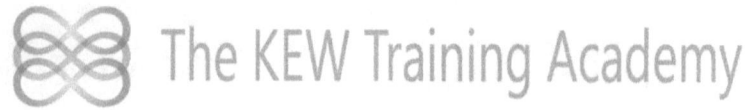

3. State it in the present tense.

Make it as if it is happening now. I have, I am, I'm doing... what are you doing right now, attending this session is a positive step forward.

4. Is it achievable and realistic?

Has someone else already achieved this or might they achieve this? Is it realistic for you? If one person can achieve something then so can you.

5. Set a time and make it an exciting outcome

There is some debate about setting a date and some people feel uncomfortable about this. If it is a small goal then do it. If it is a really big goal then I advise that you leave the time for the moment until it starts to look like things are moving.

6. Finally how will you achieve your goal?

For example

By going to the gym twice are week, going for a walk twice per week, changing certain things you eat, doing things in a manageable way to suit your lifestyle, choose exercises and activities you enjoy

Remember not to overestimate what you can achieve in a week and under estimate what can be achieved in 6 months

To be successful in anything you need to have an outcome in mind. There's the old saying you might have heard, "If you don't know where you are going, you'll end up somewhere else." This is a simple formula that allows to create well formed outcomes.

Stated positively

Always set goals in the positive sense. That is, what do you want, rather than what you don't want.

"What can you do to bring this about by your own actions?""What can you do to influence the outcome?" "What do you need to do to achieve this goal?"

Defined in sensory specific terms

.   (a) "What date do you intend to have this outcome by?"

.   (b) "Put yourself in the situation of having it. What do you see/hear/feel when you have it?" Make sure that your image of the goal is sensory-rich, vivid and compelling.

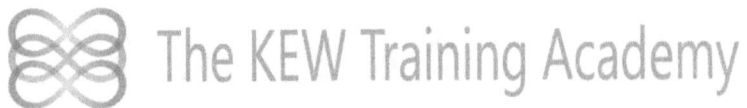

Ecology" (Effects on every area of your life)

This is a 'risk assessment' on how the goal will affect every area of your life.

"What will happen when you have it?" "What won't happen when you have it?""Are there any downsides to achieving it?"

"How would having this outcome affect each area of your life?""Who else would be affected by you having this outcome?""How would you having this outcome affect the planet?"

"How do you feel about this goal?" "Do you want it 100%?" "Does your energy increase when you think about it?" If not, adjust the goal until you feel enthusiastic about it!

Resources and Route

What resources do you have that will help you reach your goal? What additional resources do you need?

It's much easier to work out how to get to your goal once you've got there!

Put yourself in the position of having achieved the goal. What had to be in place immediately before to allow your goal to happen? And what had to be in place before that? Continue all the way back to the very first step.

Using Submodalities to help with Weight Loss

This technique can be used to help someone stop smoking, lose weight or overcome any kind of addiction, alcohol or drugs.

Six Step Reframe for Weight Loss

Reframing is the process of helping the client to develop new meanings and understandings about an unwanted behaviour. We can use this session to help the client to identify at least one internal motivation that prompts overeating or unnecessary eating (that is, eating when not really hungry).

This session works on the premise that everything that we do, we do for a reason. In NLP and Hypnotherapy one of the premises is that all parts within an individual's personality serves a positive intention – usually satisfying basic human physical and emotional needs, values and beliefs. In theory we could say then that "parts" influence actions and behaviours intended to fulfil positive intentions, even when the intentions are known only at a subconscious level.

Parts sometimes prompt unwanted or hurtful or self-harming behaviours in attempts to satisfy these positive intentions. Ironically, these hurtful behaviours often cause the very problems they are intended to prevent. Often as in the case of overeating, the positive intention may be to provide comfort or to relieve stress. Even though wolfing down a packet of chocolate biscuits can bring momentary sense of wellbeing or pleasure, the after math result of regret and disgust can be very uncomfortable, and the resulting weight gain can be a source of additional discomfort and stress.

The six step reframe helps you and the client contact the clients "part of self" responsible for overeating, identify the positive intention behind overeating or binging and persuade that part to choose alternatives to overeating.

I like to tell my clients that this is a method that takes all the energy attached to overeating and channels that energy in a new, healthier direction.

Session

Explain that the purpose of this session is to help the client identify the underlying reasons for overeating or binging.

This method enhances the clients ability to control runaway eating patterns. It helps the client examine an unwanted behaviour or habit from a new perspective, and metaphorically, to communicate with a part of self that is causing the problem behaviour.

Here are the steps. Note: For each step ask the client to close their eyes, complete the step and then open their eyes.

1. Identify the part

a. Introduce the "parts" frame.

Sometimes when people repeatedly do things they regret, or wish they didn't do, but they can't seem to stop themselves, we could say that a "part of self" is prompting the unwanted behaviour. "I want to teach you a method for contacting the part of yourself that has led you to over eat the wrong kinds of foods, identify the parts positive intention for you, and ask that part to find alternative ways to satisfy the intention, so that you can channel that energy in more positive directions."

b. Teach the client how to establish inner contact with the part.

"In a moment I'm going to ask you to relax, close your eyes and mentally invite that part into your conscious awareness, there's no right or wrong way to do this, it is an intuitive process, so just be open and receptive to your inner experience. The part will make itself known to you in one of many ways. Perhaps it will be an image in your mind, such as a symbol, an object or a memory. Or it might be something you feel on a physical level – a sensation. It might be some inner dialogue – something you say to yourself. Whatever you experience will be just fine. Now make yourself comfortable, take a deep breath, relax, close your eyes and go ahead. When you have some indication from that part, just let me know."

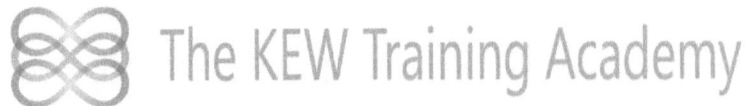

2. Establish Yes from the part. – Ideomotor Signalling or get client to talk.

Help the client establish communication with the part.

"Ask the part if it is willing to communicate with you, and let me know the answer."

3. Identify the Positive Intention

Ask the client to reconnect with the part and find out the positive intention behind overeating.

"Close your eyes and connect with the part and ask the part to tell you the positive intention behind your overeating. In other words, what does the part want to do for you by causing you to over eat? What is it trying to give to you? Just relax now and let the answers come to you. Whenever you're ready just open your eyes and let me know."

(Sometimes the clients response will indicate a very clear, logical intention. At other times the clients response is vague and seemingly irrelevant. In the latter case it is up to you to help the client flesh out the meaning of the response and figure out the positive intention. Somehow there usually is a connection)

(Sometimes the client gives a response that suggests a negative intention instead of a positive one. Your reply should be, "and what would that do for you?" Keep asking until you get a positive intention. For example a client once said to me that the intention of over eating was "to make me die". When I then asked "What would dyeing do for you?" her reply was, "So I could go to heaven and be happy". I then inquired, "Are there other ways for you to go to heaven without having to over eat? Are there other ways to be happy now, without having to wait until you die?".

4. Help the client find alternatives to satisfy the positive intention.

a. Explain to the client that parts often get stuck in a rut, using ineffective or harmful methods to satisfy a positive intention and not knowing what else to do. Tell the client that you are going to give that part instructions so that it can access the client's inner resources- such as creativity, intuition, and inner wisdom – and can consider alternatives to overeating.

"Now as you relax and reconnect with that part. It may seem the same or it may seem different somehow. We want this part to understand that overeating does not solve the problem or satisfy the positive intention, and overeating in this way is actually harmful and unhealthy. So now this part has an opportunity to do its job more effectively, with more flexibility.

Tell this part you are giving it full access to your inner resources, such as your creativity, your intuition, and your inner wisdom, so that it can begin to learn more than ever before. The part can access these inner resources right now, even as I am speaking to you. As this

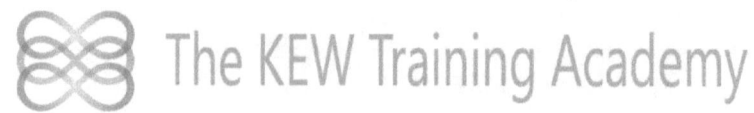

part is learning and improving, it can begin to create a list of additional ways to accomplish that positive intention – healthy, convenient ways to do it... numerous options and alternatives to overeating, so that overeating is no longer the only choice....and that energy gets channelled into more positive directions for you.

As that part of yourself begins to register all these options and alternatives, it can select three of those options and bring them into your conscious awareness for your review and approval. So when those three selections....those alternatives....are available to you....open your eyes."

b. Wait quietly while your client completes this step. When the clients eyes are open, ask about the three selections. Evaluate with the client whether these selections are realistic and suitable for satisfying the positive intention. At least one of these choices should be easy and convenient to do – offering the same ease and convenience as food. Encourage the client to appreciate the creativity that brought these selections forth and to notice how well the part is cooperating.

(Some clients do not think of 3 alternatives. They might instead think of 2 or 1 or maybe more such as 4 or 5. Whatever number they come up with, accept them and tell the client that they are doing good work.)

5. Enter into a contract with the part

a. Instruct the client to make a contract or agreement with the part to choose one of the healthier alternatives whenever there is need to fill the positive intention that led to overeating:

"Close your eyes and relax again and thank that part for selecting those alternatives. Know you have additional ways to take care of yourself and meet your needs. I ask you now to enter into a contract with that part, such that from now on, whenever you need to satisfy that intention (e.g cope with stress, boredom, comfort yourself etc) that part will automatically chose one of these healthier alternatives.

In fact should that part require even more flexibility, it can continue to access your creativity, your intuition, and your inner wisdom to arrive at additional healthy, positive choices that will serve your needs and desires.

When this part is in agreement with this contract, nod your head. On the other hand, if that part has any concerns or reservations, open your eyes and let's talk about them."

6. Future Rehearsal

a. Have the client mentally review the new alternatives to overeating:

"Close your eyes again and thank that part for entering into the contract with you. See images in which you are choosing suitable, healthy ways to take care of yourself. Step into those images one by one and enjoy the new behaviours."

b. Guide the client through possible future scenarios in which he or she is choosing one or more of the alternatives selected in step 4, in order to satisfy the positive intention. For example:

"Imagine you've come home from a hard day at work, and you want to relax and unwind and pamper yourself (the positive intention). You sit down and begin to listen to some of your favourite music or go for a walk (one of the alternatives to overeating). As you close your eyes and relax, a sense of contentment comes over you and all the cares and frustrations of the day seem to melt away and you feel so much more at ease. You are so pleased and satisfied that you have found this method of pampering yourself."

Full Weight Loss Session – Including Induction

"And as you just concentrate on your breathing and just completely let go...you start to relax...and don't try to make it happen, just let it happen... just imagine a wave of relaxation washing over your body like water in the shower going from your head down to your toes.

And I want you to picture ten steps going down, and as I count backwards from ten to one you can literally feel your feet moving onto step ten, you can see your feet making contact with step 9, you can hear your feet touching step 8 and now you're taking step 7 and 6 and just going deeper into an awareness of yourself, your taking step 5 as each muscle turns loose, lets loose and you go deeper, your taking step three as you gently calmly easily move on to an even deeper level, your taking step 2, and now you're taking step 1...

And you are just going deeper and deeper, and deeper just means going deeper into an awareness of yourself, you aren't going to be asleep this is just a sleep of the nervous system and you are going to really like it, and you can see everything, hear everything, feel everything and you are going to really enjoy just being completely relaxed...and even when you are not aware of it your brilliant mind is seeing, believing and accepting every word I'm saying, and as you go deeper into a different state of awareness you are so aware that you have a strong desire, a compelling powerful irresistible desire and ability to become slimmer, to become leaner, and this desire.... this motivating ability to become lean and slim... is becoming such a powerful... permanent part of you, that it overrules any old negative eating habits, and instead you are now constantly motivated to act in a completely different way.

You are motivated to act in a way that causes you to shed excess weight quite easily and quite healthily, and to become thinner and fitter and healthier for life, and as you go deeper your subconscious mind is remembering that you were actually born with a perfect body.... with a perfect attitude to food, as a baby you were so perfectly in tune with your body that you knew when to eat... and you knew when to stop eating... and you have never ever lost

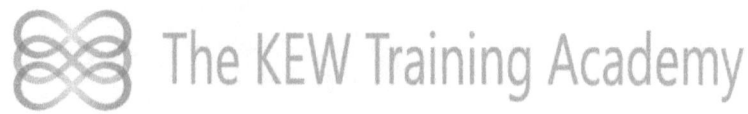
this ability, and right now you are powerfully re-activating, and re- generating that ability through the power and direction of your subconscious mind.

Your brilliant subconscious mind is reactivating, regenerating and re-manifesting in you that perfect attitude to food that you were born with and that still exists within you, and while your subconscious mind remembers that and gives it right back to you, your conscious mind is forgetting everything it needs to forget.... your remembering everything you need to remember that allows you to have a normal weight and a normal relationship to food..... and at the same time your conscious mind is forgetting any old negative habits, they are simply becoming erased, eradicated, eliminated and gone...... they are in your past now, they are all behind you and out of your life, you remember everything you need to remember with your subconscious mind to become and stay slim, and your conscious mind forgets everything you need to forget, you remember to eat when you are hungry, you automatically remember to eat slowly you remember to leave food, and then you remember to forget about food for hours afterwards, in fact you have the same attitude to eating that you have to sleeping, you remember to sleep and when you've had enough sleep you forget all about it, you remember to eat selectively and then you forget all about eating because you are becoming so perfectly in tune with your body and you and your body are working together now as a perfect team.

You respond to your body by eating healthy nutritious food that allows you to become thinner, lighter and healthier and you are so aware that you have an absolute right to be slim, a drive and a commitment to be slim, and every single day you feel powerfully motivated and conditioned to eat differently, in fact you feel so differently about food now that you see food as fuel for your body and you only want to eat the food that your body can use... you only want to eat healthy natural fresh food....

You love exercising, you always fit it into your schedule, you are now so easily happily and so willingly choosing to be thinner... and you are loving the process, you are free from self-destructive eating habits... your free forever from self-destructive self-defeating eating habits... there is no room in your mind, in your body, in your life for overeating.

From now on overeating is something you used to do, it just cannot... will not... does not influence you any longer, it is all behind you... it is in the past now... it is out of your life... as you move on from one great achievement to another... and you are moving on from one phenomenal achievement to another, you're eating so differently now and enjoying the process..... you are becoming lighter all the time and it is just so easy, you have so much more energy, you exercise willingly and you absolutely enjoy it, you love that feeling of fitting in to smaller clothes and you feel such a powerful sense of accomplishment and achievement, food could never give you that feeling that you are giving to yourself, as you take control of how you look and how you feel and how you eat, you have decided to change your weight and your shape and your size and you easily take all the action that makes this happen you are erasing and eliminating forever poor eating habits.

You find yourself easily refusing the wrong food, you find yourself happily saying no the kind of food that can only harm your body... you love your body you want to take care of it, you treat your body with respect and you chose healthy food, you eat less food automatically, you love leaving some food on your plate, you love refusing the wrong type of food it makes you feel so powerful, and as you love your body it is loving you right back... it is becoming the way you want it to be.... looking the way you want it to look... and you feel so happy... you welcome... you celebrate you enjoy the good restrictions you are making , you absolutely delight in leaving food and throwing it away, I want you to see yourself in your mind right now at your ideal weight, just feel how lean you are, you can feel the difference there's less of you, you can hear people praising you telling you "you look amazing"....

And you are amazing because you are doing this for yourself, you can hear people praising you, noticing all of the achievements and you notice how much happier your body is now that you respect it... you like it, you want to do things that keep it in a healthy attractive state, so make an image of how you want to look and you can see it very clearly... you can see yourself leaner lighter, you might prefer to feel like there's less of you as you do up your jeans or your waist band, you might want to hear people telling you that you need a different size in a shop, you can use all your senses, see yourself as leaner lighter wearing all the clothes you've always wanted to wear, looking and feeling the way you've always wanted to look, hearing people tell you how great you look, feeling yourself wearing a smaller size and you particularly notice that your body just feels so good because you respect it... you like it...

You want to do the right things for it... and as you focus on this image, seeing feeling hearing how good you look as you focus on this image using all of your senses, you are moving towards this image right now, because your inner mind is picking up that your strongest desire is to reach and maintain this desired shape and weight, your strongest desire is to choose to be thinner, fitter, stronger and healthier, to welcome... to celebrate the exciting changes you are making and you absolutely know that you are enough... of course you are enough... you are always enough.... you are more than enough... you remind yourself of this absolute truth every day many times every day, just after you wake up... just before you go to bed, at the beginning and end of every meal you remind yourself... I am enough... and as you repeat this absolute truth to yourself you find yourself needing less food... you are enough, you have enough and now that you know with unshakable certainty that you are enough you need less food all the time it is all so easy... you are now and forever a selective moderate eater... those negative habits have gone forever they are just fading shrinking disappearing gone, leaving you free to eat the way you were put on the planet to eat...

In a healthy normal way leaving you slimmer, fitter, more attractive and happier, your inner mind the most powerful healing force there is, is releasing you... freeing you... from any old habits, you are moving so far, far, far away from overeating, you can literally feel it shrinking disappearing, going gone.... it is out of your life forever and you celebrate you rejoice you welcome its absence... and now that you eat differently for life your body is becoming a more efficient machine, using all the healthy calories that you take in to build a perfect

Hypnotherapy Practitioner Course - Professional Accredited Hypnotherapy Training

healthy body for you, you nourish your body with natural fruit and vegetables with real healthy food and you find yourself wanting and eating less, and while you're eating less your metabolic rate is increasing through the power and direction of your inner mind, right now just feel and believe and imagine your metabolic rate working as perfectly as it did when you were a child... when you were a little baby you had a perfect super- efficient metabolism... and you are regaining that right now... because your mind and body know, they know how to speed your metabolic rate up, to make it work as perfectly as it did when you were a new-born and as you think about that you are literally causing it to happen... because every thought you think creates a physical reaction...

Your thinking about remembering reactivating coming into this world with a perfect metabolic rate and your metabolic rate is super-efficient... and your stomach is so tiny your stomach is the size of a fist... so right now just take your fist and squeeze it... and just repeat to yourself in your imagination in your head, my stomach is the size of my fist, my stomach is the size of my fist, my stomach is the size of my fist, and you might even notice the feeling of your stomach shrinking right now, you might even notice the feeling of your stomach contracting becoming smaller right now as you concentrate on this feeling through the power and direction of your inner mind, your stomach is becoming small, your stomach is becoming tiny, and you automatically find yourself eating enough food to satisfy that capacity of a fist and then stopping quite easily, stopping naturally and automatically simply because you want to, you squeeze your fist before every meal to remind yourself that you are enough and that you can and you will be the best that you can be, you squeeze your fist before every meal to remind yourself that you have a small stomach and you find yourself continuously constantly confidently wanting and eating less food, you enjoy the food you eat but you just want and need less of it, from now on you eat only in response to real hunger, whenever you feel hungry you will ask yourself on a scale of 1-10 just how hungry am I? And you will only ever eat when you are at an 8 on that scale...you will now only eat in response to real hunger...

You are now and forever a sensible and selective eater... you stay away from wheat products and fatty foods...you see your body as a fine race horse...this race horse can and will win you many races in life...but to look after your winning racehorse you must only feed it the finest healthiest ingredients.... you now drink lots of water every day to assist your body in eliminating excess waste, you crave water, you drink 8 glasses every day your skin is glowing you just feel fabulous, you drink some water as soon as you wake up you are automatically drinking water and you are automatically leaving some food at every meal, you love that feeling of choice, you love that feeling of choosing to leave a little something, and you always chose to leave something as it makes you feel so powerful, it makes you feel like you are in control and you always will be, food cannot control you because you are taking charge of how you eat, how you look how you feel, you have such a positive attitude to your body , you have an overwhelming positive focused drive to become and to stay slim for good, and you are changing your language and your focus, you are changing your beliefs your whole relationship with food for the better and your body is changing quite easily because of this.

Hypnotherapy Practitioner Course - Professional Accredited Hypnotherapy Training

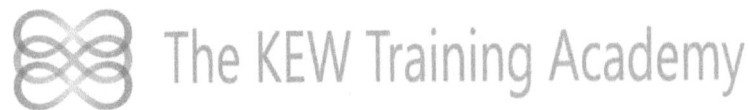

I will now count you back from 1 to 10, and on the sound of 10 you will be fully re-charged, full of energy, vitality with an overwhelming sense of positivity and motivation to reach all your goals....

1, 2, 3, 4, 5, 6, 7, 8, 9, 10...........

Easy Weight Loss Script

Drifting down now into a very deep and comfortable relaxation - your subconscious mind is in the ideal state for visualization and suggestions - and even though you've felt uncomfortable with your weight for a while now - you are able to remember a time when you were just the ideal weight and shape for your height - and if you've never been that ideal weight it really doesn't matter - because your creative subconscious mind can imagine how it will feel - when you've lost those excess pounds - to be able to move easily and freely - without the burden of carrying around all of the excess weight.

And I'm sure that you know what I mean - feeling excess weight around the buttocks and the thighs - feeling sluggish and hardly able to move - in the comfortable and easy way that your body knows how - being unable to wear all those wonderful clothes that you know would look so good on a slimmer body - having less energy than you'd like - these are not good feelings for you - so far you have endured them - perhaps dreading stepping onto those scales and watching how the pounds have been steadily creeping up and up - knowing that sooner or later you'd have to do something about it - but putting off the inevitable - until now.

Well - now - you've decided that it's time to revert to that slimmer and healthier you - and because you've decided - because you've already got it into your mind that now is the time - you're going to find that weight loss is easy - and you're going to lose that excess weight – quite easily as the weeks go bye - your lifestyle is changing now - even - especially - as you drift deeper and deeper into this comfortable and relaxing state.

The first thing that your mind is beginning to accept is that in order to lose weight you are going to be burning off more calories than you take in - so - no matter what you have eaten or drunk on a daily basis in the past - you are going to find that you now no longer need or want to eat or drink nearly as much - if you've ever snacked in between meals than you no longer feel that you want to do that - your appetite is reducing and you no longer think of food in the way that you used to do.

When you do eat - you do so to live - you no longer live to eat - you eat to live - food is just a necessary and sometime inconvenient distraction to whatever else is going on around you. You do find however that you have no desire for sweet, fatty or otherwise unhealthy food or drink - you concentrate instead of feeding your body with the healthy nutrients that it needs.

You find that there is always something better to do than to eat - and you're eating less and less each and every day - simply because food isn't an important part of your life. Your mind is focused elsewhere - your pastimes - your relationships - your zest for living - whatever is important for you as the wonderful, creational person that you are.

From this moment on you begin to enjoy using your body to its maximum potential - and if you're a driver and enjoyed driving your car or even being driven from place to place you now really prefer to walk - you make a determined effort to walk whenever you can - whether it is up and down stairs - to the shops - into town - or to visit friends - it really doesn't matter - the fact is that walking is becoming very important to you.

You find that you can not only double - but treble your walking distance - and even when time is of essence - you so much prefer to walk. It reminds you that you really are now losing weight - losing weight and feeling wonderful. Losing weight and feeling great.

During your walks your mind begins to find so many different things to concentrate on - any problems that you've been experiencing during your everyday life are resolved on an unconscious level by your wonderful, creative subconscious mind - and you walk - and you walk as much as is possible for you - depending upon your daily circumstances and your lifestyle.

You have more energy during your normal, everyday activities and find yourself up and on the go - as much as you can - no more sitting around doing nothing at all - that's not for you - and even as you begin moving around more and more - you're aware that this is the way that it's meant to be - so natural to you - as a human being with legs and arms you are meant to exercise and utilize your body - to burn off the excess fat - rather than sitting and stagnating like a saggy aged old vegetable that's ready for the bin.

The benefit for you in this exercise is that you not only have more energy and more vitality - but you really do begin to lose weight - to become slimmer and healthier - fitter and so much more motivated too - to lose that excess weight - and the wonderful thing is that it's so easy for you - because this is the way that you were meant to be.

So - if you will - imagine yourself now at the weight and size that you've set your mind on. See yourself - slimmer - healthier - fitter and so much more confident - knowing that you look and feel so good. See what you're wearing - don't those clothes look so good on your wonderful, slim and healthy body? How do you feel? Imagine the congratulations and praises that people are giving you for losing that fat - but - it is nowhere near as important to you as how you feel about yourself - right now - you are slim, you are healthy, you are your ideal weight - and size for your height - you look good - you feel good - you are good. This is your ideal self - so - take the image of your ideal self and place it up there in your mind - to remind - over and over again - how good it will be when you've lost that excess weight.

You may find that there are days when you just don't feel like walking - that's fine if it's just the odd day - but - if your body is physically fit and healthy then you'll find that - by the following day - your determination and motivation will have doubled - because you'll just want to catch up - because you really can't wait to lose that excess weight.

And - if your body isn't physically fit and healthy - that's not such a problem - you will pace yourself - becoming in touch with your body and knowing what it is capable of is important to you - you will push yourself only as far as you know you can safely go - realizing perhaps that a little further - will come with time - and it will - you're unconscious mind will let you know when it's time to stop - and there is a time to stop - and a time to go - and you're on the go so much more - as you move toward your healthier, slimmer self.

And these suggestions are firmly embedded in your subconscious mind and grow stronger and stronger day by day. Stronger by the day, stronger by the hour, stronger by the minute.

So in a moment- when you're ready - I'm going to count from one to five and at the count of five you'll be wide awake.

One, two, three, four, five.

Car Weight Loss Script

Begin with an Induction and Deepener

You have come to a point in your life where you are ready to rid yourself of eating in response to emotions. You have tried it in the past and it has not worked. At the very best, eating may have distracted you from your emotions but then the emotion came back again. There is no food, sweets or drink, that could ever satisfy any emotion that you have ever experienced. You tried that and it has not worked.

All of your feelings are good. All of your feelings are there for a reason. There is no difference between the five outer senses, touch, taste, sight, smell and hearing, and all of your inner emotions that we call feelings. They are there to help you, to protect you and to guide you, so that you can take care of yourself in a way that is most beneficial to you.

Your feelings are like the gauges and lights on the dash board of a car. These lights and gauges on the car are there for a reason. They help you to know what to do in order to keep it running efficiently so that it will run reliably for a long time. This allows you to get the most out of your car. The best performance and value. The same goes for you and your body... feelings help tell you how to take the best care of yourself.

If you treated a car the way you have been treating your body, the car would soon be in trouble, much the same way that you are in trouble now from overeating. When the oil light, lights up in a car, the driver does not pull into a petrol station and put more petrol into the tank, especially if the tank is already full. This is what you have been doing to your body.

You are here because, in the past when you felt a feeling such as anxiety, frustration, boredom, depression, or whatever it may be, and you have tried to feed that feeling. You know this is true, because you have tried it and it did not work.

When the oil light on a car goes on, it indicates that the driver needs to check the oil.

When the temperature light goes on, the driver needs to check the water in the radiator.

When the wind shield wiper fluid light goes on, the driver needs to put in more fluid, and so on. These lights are good. They need to be attended too. Putting more gas in the car will not help any of these situations.

When you feel anxious, it is a signal, to look around, something in your life needs fixing.

When you feel depressed, it is a signal, to become more effective. It's a call to action.

When you feel frustrated, it is a signal, that what you are doing is not working, try something else.

When you feel stressed out, it means that you are trying to do too much, to do it all well, you need to do something else to help you relax.

When you feel loneliness, it means that you have a healthy desire for human contact. Call someone, write a letter, check your e-mail, join a club, or become a volunteer.

Eating does not satisfy any of these feelings any more than putting more petrol in your car will fix an oil or temperature problem. I want your subconscious mind to now give you an alternative to eating for when you become stressed, or frustrated or bored or are feeling any kind of emotion....let the power of your subconscious mind show you now as the new you...., either joining a club........**(enter new alternatives as discussed)**

Now you will find it easier to know what each of your feelings are trying to indicate for you to do. As you can now see, all of your feelings are good. Just as good as the five senses. They are there to guide you ad protect you. Somewhere you got the wires crossed. Now we are correcting that.

The reason your wires might have gotten crossed is because some time ago, probably when you were very young, you felt a feeling and you could not act in response to it. You had the feeling, but try as you might, because of your circumstances, could do little or nothing about what was causing the feeling.

So even if you did understand what the feeling was trying to tell you, there was little you could do about it. You wound up forgetting what the feeling even meant for you to do. You

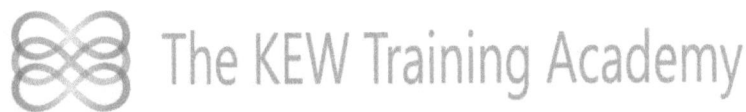

then mistakenly found temporary comfort in the distraction of food. It didn't really help. But there was more food, and more feelings, and you fell into that rut. Now you are climbing out of that rut.

You are now ready, to begin a life that is much more satisfying than the one you have been living. Now you are capable of satisfying yourself like never before.

Now, when a feeling comes up again, you'll know what to do. In fact you will begin to look forward to acting upon your feelings in a more satisfying way. For example, if you feel lonely, you can call a friend, visit someone, or go to a place where you can meet people. Loneliness can never be satisfied with food. You now understand that to be a fact.

And just as loneliness cannot be satisfied by food, neither can stress, frustration, anxiety, depression, boredom, or any other feeling.

You are now free from the frustrating cycle that has caused you so much distress and weight gain. From this moment onwards, you will eat only when you are sure that you need re-fuelling and you will ask yourself on a scale of 1-10....just how hungry am I? And you will only eat when you are at an 8 on that scale and you are sure that your body really does need refuelling and that you are not just trying to feed an emotion. You will now begin to satisfy yourself in many new and more interesting and fulfilling ways rather than food. From now on when you get a feeling, and it is not hunger, you will simply say, STOP, this is important, I'm giving this my 100% effort. My feelings are trying to tell me something important. Then listen to the feeling, and begin to act on it.

I want you to concentrate on all of the wonderful things that makes you unique, that makes you the very special unique person that you are now. And you might take this opportunity to focus on how you can improve on the things in your life that you would like to improve.

Gastric Band Session 1 – Initial Session

This is a set the scene type script...the initial session at the hospital to gather information before the operation takes place, use after an induction and deepener...

As you drift even more deeply into this deep hypnotic sleep...so comfortable...so relaxing...I'm going to take you on an imaginative journey whereby you can use the power of your wonderful subconscious mind to help you to get rid of the excess weight that you have been carrying around for so long. And it's because you really want to get rid of that weight that you have decided to use Gastric Band in hypnosis to help you...you have heard or read of the success stories of others who have reduced their weight by this method...the surgery is non-invasive and has excellent results.

Hypnosis-Gastric-Band surgery is even safer because you can undergo this operation without physically going 'under the knife'. Therefore, I need you to listen very carefully and allow your sub- conscious to visualize or become aware of everything I suggest to the very best of your ability...make the images real...notice any sounds or smells that accompany your impressions.

Pause...Firstly...imagine that you have chosen the hospital where your procedure is to take place and you are in the surgeons/consultants office...undergoing your first consultation. (Good idea to use some hospital smells here, waft some antiseptic) The consultant is friendly, you shake hands and immediately you feel at ease. Your consultant explains that obesity isn't something to be ashamed of...it is a dis-order which can be treated successfully by using this method. You listen carefully as the doctor provides you with all the facts. You will have the operation by keyhole surgery which will take about one hour under a general anaesthetic and there will be no side effects, no discomfort. There will be follow- up appointments a few weeks apart when you will decide if the band needs to be adjusted. You really want to go through with this surgery...you can't wait to be rid of this excess weight and you leave the clinic knowing this is the right course of action for you, feeling happy and optimistic. Soon your stomach will be the size of a golf ball and you will be happy eating smaller portions of healthy nutritional food. Clothes that you never thought you would wear become reality. (Finish as you think appropriate)

Gastric Band Session Two...The operation

Now it is the day for your operation, the day you have been waiting for has arrived. Picture and imagine yourself preparing for the journey to the hospital and now let's go in the taxi/car/bus (Check this beforehand for authenticity) and see yourself arrive at the hospital. Walking in through the main doors and following the signs for your ward. See yourself checking in at reception, the receptionist smiles and gives you reassurance, telling you how good your chosen consultant is.

You follow her to your room and a nurse enters and checks your name. You are asked to get changed into the hospital gown and await your pre-op preparation. As you sit comfortably in your chair the door opens and in comes your nurse to prepare you for surgery. You lie on the bed and the nurse does everything necessary to prepare you for surgery, checking blood pressure and temperature and makes some notes on your sheet. She puts a hospital bracelet onto your wrist before leaving the room. Then she leaves you to relax. You have not eaten or drunk anything, fasting since the night before and yet surprisingly not feeling hungry. After a short time, the door opens and a man in a blue gown enters your room. He introduces himself to you as the anaesthetist, asks a few questions and explains what is going to happen.

He is followed by your consultant who gives you a few tips about what to expect and gives you a general run through on the operating procedure. The gastric band operation usually takes about an hour and he is going to use keyhole surgery as previously explained. During your operation a number of small incisions will be made in your abdomen (Tummy), rather than one large cut. Then he will make four to five small cuts on your upper abdomen using very small instruments, guided by a laparoscope (a long, thin telescope with a light and camera lens at the tip), to place the band around the top part of your stomach. Then the band is connected to the injection port, which is placed just under the skin.

Then he will lock it in place so that it can't come undone. Afterwards, the cuts are closed with two or three dissolvable stitches.....

The gastric band contains a circular balloon which can be filled with saline and this will be used to adjust your band after your operation. You will need to rest after your operation and be able to go home the next day. None of this bothers you as you are just pleased to be having the operation and you thank him for taking the time to explain this. Then he says that they will provide you with healthy eating guides and information on different activities, which will be beneficial for you.

The healthy eating guides won't be an issue for you because you won't want to eat junk foods and you won't be able to overeat...the gastric band will make sure of that. The consultant leaves and shortly afterwards it is time to be taken to the operating theatre. The trolley arrives and you are gently eased onto it, and covered with a sheet. As you lie flat on the trolley, you hear the sound of nurses talking, going about their daily routines (Play sound effect here) all you can see are the overhead lights as you move down the corridor and into the lift, down to the operating theatre. As you are wheeled into the theatre you recognise the antiseptic smell which to you indicates cleanliness (Waft some antiseptic now).

The anaesthetist greets you...part of his face is covered but you recognize those twinkling eyes... he asks for your name and your date of birth as he prepares your injection and gently rubs the area with a swab of cotton wool and some cool liquid and inserts the Cannula to flow in the anaesthetic. A nurse is on the other side of you...she is holding your hand and talking to you as though she had known you all your life..."Can you feel anything?" the anaesthetist enquires as he gently prods your stomach...and you realize that the area is numb and you answer no nothing at all...Even with the bright lights overhead you are beginning to feel a little drowsy... sleepy...and close your eyes. The surgeon is now ready to perform the keyhole surgery and he explains that you will feel no discomfort at all and the nurse tells you that everything's going fine....just as it should. The surgeon is very skilled and knows exactly what he's doing. His white gloved hands are gentle and you feel so comfortably relaxed that you now begin to drift off...into a deep, comfortable sleep...I'll be quiet for a few moments whilst you drift into this wonderful, peaceful sleep.....

...and as you sleep your operation is started and you do not feel any of the incisions as they are so small...you do not feel the camera going in as it is all so gentle and you are in a deep hypnotic type sleep. It is completed safely using the keyhole method just as was explained to you by your consultant. Time has no meaning and the one hour could have been three as it was all so pleasant.

Pause...After a while, you open your eyes and look around...wondering at first where you are...then realise you are back in your hospital room...and you remember...your Gastric Band surgery...Once you are back on solids you notice you are eating slowly and really chewing your food well before swallowing. You find you are placing you're eating utensils down between bites because you eat so slowly...This is good because it gives you a chance to savour and enjoy each mouthful...and because you are easily full, you find that you can't eat anywhere near as much as you used to do...Pause...The anaesthetic has started to wear off a little and you notice now where the keyhole surgery was performed...there is a slight discomfort...yet it's easily bearable and you know it will soon wear off. The nurse arrives and takes your temperature once more...before checking your blood pressure again. A drip is inserted to give you fluids until the anaesthetic is completely gone. She tells you that everything's fine...and the operation went well...just as you knew it would. You rest now for a couple of hours...and the nurse returns and does your health checks before removing the drip just in time...as the drinks trolley arrives and you are asked what you would like to drink. You sip it slowly...thankful for the refreshing liquid. You are encouraged to get up and sit in the chair next to your bed. You feel so glad that you have had the surgery and can't wait to get rid of the excess weight.....

As you sip your drink the nurse gives you some advice about caring for your healing wounds and informs you that the surgeon used dissolvable stitches and it is likely they will disappear in about seven to ten days' time. She also reminds you that a general anaesthetic temporarily affects your co-ordination and reasoning skills and you must not drive or drink alcohol or sign any legal documents for 48 hours after today. You understand that you will need to make major changes to your eating habits and make different choices in the future. Initially you will have only liquids before moving onto pureed food and you might need to take vitamin supplements. After a while, your first nutritional liquid (meal) arrives. You think to yourself that this will never satisfy my appetite...however...

Amazingly...after just a few sips... you find that you are already full...It's the same with every pureed meal you eat...you drink or sup this pureed food and find that you are surprisingly full. Finding that you are so easily satisfied that you just don't want any more food. The next few hours go by in a haze...until it's time for you to be discharged. Your consultant has been back to visit you and is pleased with how everything went.

You are given an appointment for a follow up check and told that your (Husband/wife/son) is here to take you home...You are now dressed and your bag is packed. You say thanks to the nurses who cared so well for you as prepare to leave...

Pause...Over the next few days and weeks...once you are back on solids you notice you are eating slowly and really chewing your food well before swallowing. You find you are placing you're eating utensils down between bites because you eat so slowly...This is good because it gives you a chance to savour and enjoy each mouthful...and because you are easily full,

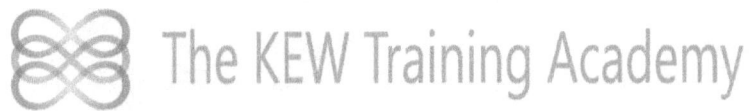
you find that you can't and do not want to eat anywhere near as much as you used to do...you find yourself eating very small portions of healthy, nutritious food. The memory of the operation soon wears off and you are getting back into the swing of everyday life and you find that you are able to do all the things that you used to do...much more easily now...

The excess weight is dropping off you...you are becoming lighter and slimmer and happier and proud of yourself. Your confidence increases day by day...and you realize that it's all down to your gastric band operation...Pause...In a moment, I'm going to count you out of hypnosis...you will feel exactly as though this operation occurred in your physical life...The memory of the surgery will remain vivid and clear.

In a moment, I am going to count from one to five and on five you will come back to full conscious awareness (Therapist speak with more feeling and conviction)

Feeling wonderfully relaxed...Feeling Wonderfully Good... Physically...Mentally...and Emotionally feeling better than you have felt for Days...Weeks...Perhaps even Months...Re-energized and alert...

(Therapist start counting now)...Number One...slowly coming back to full conscious awareness feeling wonderfully relaxed...(Therapist increase tempo)...Two...You're feeling good from head to toe...Three...Your whole body becoming alert...Four...Your eyes feel like they are bathed in spring water, your eyes begin to sparkle...And on the next number...Five...Eyes open

(Therapist click fingers on the words, Eyes open, for effect if you wish,)...WIDE AWAKE...that's right...take a deep breath and stretch.

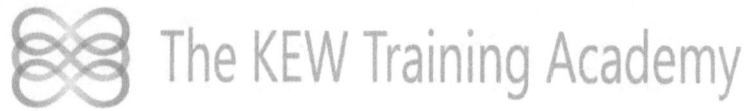

Magic of Metaphors

Hypnotherapy and Metaphors

The simplest way to deliver a metaphor is by Story Telling. A story can be understood at face value or it can be understood metaphorically, as carrying some other meaning. A metaphor always contains at least two parts: the thing stated and the thing compared to, and communicates on at least two levels: the surface meaning, and the deep structure meaning, the symbolic meaning.

In general terms, a metaphor is something that stands for something else. Metaphors can be verbal or nonverbal. Verbal metaphors can be open and obvious, for **example "*I feel like I'm dragging a great weight around with me*"**or they can be embedded in language and hidden in sensory expressions such as "*I don't know why I keep punishing myself this way*". Or they can be expressions of abstract concepts "*I feel a pain in my soul*". Nonverbal metaphors include 'body' expressions such as body language, posture, dress, sounds, gestures, lines of sight. Nonverbal also includes 'artistic' communication such as painting, writing, music, dance, play, drama, ritual and many others. Every method of communication has its own form of metaphor. Metaphor is used extensively in hypnotherapy.

Metaphor lies at the heart of all human thinking and language. Metaphor determines how we think about ourselves and how we experience the world. Metaphor shapes societies and cultures. The ability to understand one thing in terms of another is a fundamental property of being human. In therapy metaphor serves many crucial functions.

A therapist can use metaphor to:

- Invite the listener to view the world in new ways

- Enable learning & new knowledge

- Guide thinking and behaviour

- Invite active participation

- Bypass self-defeating beliefs

Metaphor plays a central role in passing on cultural values. Stories, myths and parables allow the individual to draw conclusions about how to act and how to understand their world.

In clinical practice the therapist carries on this tradition. The therapist tells a hypnotised client a story incorporating one or more carefully constructed metaphors. The client's unconscious mind then examines the metaphor for parallels in their own life. Over the next days and weeks the client will unconsciously apply the insights and reframing inherent in the

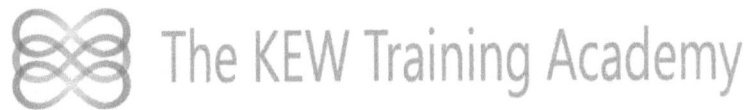

metaphor to cause changes in their own behaviour or beliefs. Metaphor therapy is therefore a form of indirect suggestion.

However, modern approaches to metaphor therapy do not stop at indirect suggestion. Some therapies supply a metaphor and ask the client to modify the metaphor to match their own mental model. Other techniques work directly on the client's own metaphors.

The basic steps to generate a metaphor for helping someone to resolve a problem or have more choices are as follows:

Identify the present situation or issue and the desired state or outcome:

Present state

Complex issue, hard to understand

Problem

Unhelpful emotion in an audience e.g. suspicion

No choices

Desired state

Simple image that everyone can make sense of and remember

Solution
Helpful emotion e.g. curiosity

Choices available

1. Notice the significant people/places/things in the situation, and the relationships between them.

2. Keeping the desired state in mind, up from the present state to a category: What is this situation/issue an example of?

3. What is another example of this category of situation or issue that includes the possibility of ending up in the desired state? Find analogies for the significant people/places/things and for the relationships between them. In the jargon, the metaphor should be 'isomorphic' with the real situation; in other words, the structure of the relationships between the elements, and the logic of the whole, should be the same, even though the content may be quite different.

The KEW Training Academy

For example, John Grinder uses the example of coaching a business owner who is engaged in a dispute with a former business partner over the ownership of a business. All of the business guy's energy is going into the dispute, and he's neglecting all sorts of other opportunities that would actually make him more money. So in Grinder's example, you might use a story about two hummingbirds fighting over a flower, while taking no notice of all the other flowers all around them.

Notice that you don't resolve the story for them - you don't talk about the two hummingbirds making up, or one of them flying away and getting loads more nectar from the other flowers. The possibilities are there, and you leave it to the person's unconscious mind to find the best possibilities for them - which may include some choice, action or idea that you hadn't thought of.

Also, keep the elements in the story relevant; one of the business people might be married, but unless the spouse was also a significant player in the situation, you wouldn't start talking about one of the hummingbirds sharing a nest.

Ideally, the metaphor will appeal to the values or interests of the listener, to keep them engaged. So the hummingbird metaphor will work best with someone who is interested in ornithology, or who is looking forward to a tropical holiday.

5. Tell the story (or mention the metaphor) and notice the response you get. You can anchor problem states and resources within the story using voice tone, facial expression or even touch. Memorable images within the story can become anchors for resources.

Where you are just coming up with a metaphor to help someone understand a complex situation, rather than for coaching or therapy purposes, you can simplify this process a bit - just ask yourself "What is this situation like?" This question leads you to chunk sideways - your unconscious mind will handle the 'chunking up' and 'chunking down to another example' steps, and you will know if you have a good example if it feels right.

Metaphors don't have to be longwinded - as little as one word in the right place may evoke a symbol with a wealth of meaning attached.

Hypnotherapy Metaphor

Your mind is like a complex network of pipes, with each pipe having its own function and route. Some pipes are interconnected, and some pipes run on their own; some pipes are very small, and some pipes are extremely well hidden. In order for the network to run efficiently, all these pipes need to be kept in good working order; occasionally polished, or repaired, or even replaced. Most of the time, you can take care of your own plumbing, ensuring that it flows freely, by giving it a bit of a clean every now and then. Sometimes though, something happens that is beyond your ability to cope, and you need to call in a plumber to prevent the network from collapsing.

Think of your hypnotherapist as that plumber. The hypnotherapist's job is to ensure that your psychological pipework is flowing well, by cleaning and unblocking the pipe; sometimes replacing pipes that have been worn away, or repairing those that are leaking. It may be necessary for your hypnotherapist to go on a search to find a hidden and elusive pipe that is proving to be irksome. You may find that your hypnotherapist has to look at old plans of the pipework with you; or perhaps help you plan a new way to run those pipes. Whatever the job, your hypnotherapist is there to help you return the network to normal or even improve it in some way or other. In order to do this properly, just like any plumber, your hypnotherapist uses and impressive array of tools.

Therapeutic Metaphors

The Philosopher and The King

Metaphors are a powerful tool in order to embed important messages into patient's unconscious minds. At different points in the treatment process certain messages need to be planted for different reasons. The following story helps show patients that they do have a choice to live or die:

Once there was a king who had a wise philosopher living in his kingdom. The king hated the philosopher because, every time the king wanted to trick the philosopher and make him look like a fool, the philosopher turned the tables and made the king look like a fool. This time the king hit upon an idea to trick the philosopher so the king could have him killed.

The king commanded, "Bring me my philosopher." The guard brought in this old man with a long white beard.

"How can your humble servant be of assistance to you, oh mighty king?" asked the philosopher.

"See this?" the king shot back, showing the old man a tiny bird in the middle of his palm. The king folded his hand around the bird and put it behind his back.

"Now, wise philosopher," the king growled at the philosopher, "is the bird alive or dead?"

The philosopher thought fast. If he said "alive" the king would squeeze the bird to death and then kill the philosopher. If he said "dead" the king would show him the bird lived and would kill him.

The philosopher thought deeply for a long moment. A smile broke out on his face and the old man said, "As you wish, great king. The result will be whatever the king wishes."

From the book "Ericksonian Approaches"

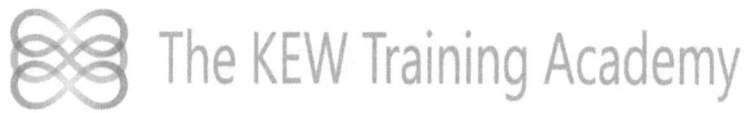
Self Appreciation

I remember about a month ago when Jimmy, my neighbour's son came to me asking if I would take him to the upcoming auto show. He was fatherless, and enjoyed watching me rebuild old collectable cars in my driveway.

As we walked the isles at the show we passed by one parked car with a bumper sticker that said "Don't touch me, I am not that kind of car". Jimmy was wondering what kind of a car it was? For one thing - this car must think highly of itself. The car didn't look much different than any other car, but after reading the sticker one would begin to wonder about the unique qualities of that particular car, and come to think of it - every car is a unique car. The cars may look alike, I said to Jimmy, as the flowers in the field look alike and the trees in the park, yet if we really pay attention we will become aware of a certain personality that attracts us to a particular car, or a flower or a tree in the park.

Just like that tree in my garden Jimmy, which I took for granted, yet the tree knew it was unlike any other. What made this tree particularly different is that it was aware of love. This tree loved itself and wanted to share its love with the world. Silently the tree sent love to the sun and the sun's rays played with the tree's branches, making it look ever more beautiful. The birds would come and perch themselves on the tree's branches, singing beautiful songs. The neighbours began to admire the tree and soon the tree seemed to be so involved in various activities and delighted that it could make others happy while enjoying itself, that it almost forgot about me ... well, that's when my eyes opened and I realized what a jewel I had in my garden.

A tree so unique, like that car right there. And you know I bet a lot of people would be so green for that car, yet they have their own special car. Just like that car there, and that one over there Jimmy ... all special cars ... to feel so good about.

So when you find me working in my driveway, fine tuning, or rebuilding my neighbour's car, I can help you choose the tools, to fix and fine tune yours ... your special car.

The Art Collection

Metaphor for smoking & substance abuse etc.

I am remembering a man I knew many years ago, called Henry, who was very interested in art. He didn't have much money, but he worked hard and saved what he could to put together a very fine collection or works of art which he was justifiably proud.

He consulted an acquaintance of his, an acknowledged expert, as to the best way of looking after his collection of fine porcelain and china. The acquaintance sold him a special substance, which he had formulated, with precise instructions as to the manner and the frequency with which it should be used. He told Henry that, if he used it regularly, then he would have no need to worry and that he could just relax, happy in the knowledge that he was doing the best he could to preserve his collection of fine works.

Henry paid the money and, throughout the years, he cleaned and lavished attention on his valued collection, always ensuring that he purchased a good supply of the compound, feeling relaxed with the thought and the idea that he was doing the best that he could to ensure the wellbeing of his works of art.

He failed to notice the fact that he always seemed to have a dull throbbing headache. The skin on his hands became reddened and sore, his fingernails became brittle and unsightly, and nothing seemed to make it better. He was unaware of the pungent smell that has become part of his person. It clung to his clothes and his hair. At least he had his collection of fine works of art.

In a few years before he managed to put aside enough money to take the holiday that he had planned for so long. Before he left, he asked a very good friend of his to look after his collection whilst he was away. He gave precise instructions as to how the art treasures should be cleaned and attended to, using the special compound that was so important for him for his peace of mind.

The friend promised to do as Henry asked, even though the smell of the compound was disgusting, and it so easily stained his hands and clothing.

Henry went on his holiday and was amazed to discover that after just a few days the headaches and the pains, the redden and sore hands, cleared up and he felt so much better and more alive than he had felt in such a long time.

Imagine how he felt on his return when he found that his friend was unwell, suffering as he had done. And the smell now so apparent upon him was disgusting. He quickly realised that the compound that he had relied on so much for peace of mind was full of poisonous and toxic chemicals. That very day Henry destroyed his whole stock of the compound, and he knew that his health was worth more than any possession no matter how valuable or rare. Henry sought further advice from the most respected experts in their field to find alternatives to look after his works of art in a healthy manner.

To his surprise, the answer was simple and inexpensive, and it had been there in front of him all the time, simple solutions of mild and appropriate cleaning materials would achieve exactly the results that he desired. His works of art would be cleaned and cared for in the most natural way that would prove healthy and beneficial.

The manufacturer of the compound would continue to produce and sell his lethal poison without regard or pity for those who would suffer from his irresponsible and mercenary actions, but Henry had made the decision to take responsibility for his own life and his own health. No longer would he rely on the advice of others whose best interests were not Henrys. He had accepted the evidence as it was, relying on his own judgement and his own ability, not knowing or needing to know how his own inner mind knew what to do for him, and I wonder now if you will not now allow your own wise inner advisor to do those things needed for you...and you will, will you not?

Continue with a Stop Smoking script after this metaphor

Metaphor – Switches for Pain

Now, before you wake up completely, I would like you to just close your eyes again and allow that drifting down again, entering again that place of calm relaxation, because there was a young boy on TV not long ago, who had learned to control all of his pain. He described the steps that he went down in his mind, one at a time down those steps, until he found this hall at the bottom, like a long tunnel, and all along this tunnel on both sides were many different switches and switchboxes, all clearly labelled. One for the right hand, one for the left, one for each leg, a switch for every part of the body, and he could see clearly the wires that carried the sensations from one place to another, all going through those switches.

All he needed to do here was to reach up in his mind and turn off the switches that he wanted to, and then he could feel nothing at all, no sensation could get through from there, because he had turned off the appropriate switches there.

He used his minds abilities differently from the man who simply made his body numb. He didn't know how he did it exactly. All he knew was, he relaxed and disconnected from the rest, moved his mind away from his body, moved it outside somewhere else, where he could watch and listen, but drift off somewhere else entirely. It really doesn't matter how you tell your subconscious what to do, or how your unconscious does it for you.

The only thing of importance is that you know you can lose sensations as easily as closing your eyes, and drifting down within where something unknown happens that allows you to disconnect, that allows that numbness to occur, and then a drifting back upwards now, towards the surface, and slowly opening the eyes as wakeful awareness returns with a comfortable continuation of that feeling of safe, secure relaxation and an ability to forget an arm, or anything at all, with no need to pay attention to things that are just fine, that somebody else can take care of for a while, while you drift in your mind and then return when it is time to enjoy that comfortable drifting upwards where the eyes open and wakeful awareness returns completely....NOW.

Introduction to Hypnotic Language Patterns

Hypnotic language patterns are not about hypnosis, because people think traditional hypnosis is about having people close their eyes and go into a trance. What hypnotic language patterns are really about is learning and harnessing the powers of our language.

These language patterns are called hypnosis because people learned about them by watching and studying with the master hypnotist Milton Erickson. One day, after they had

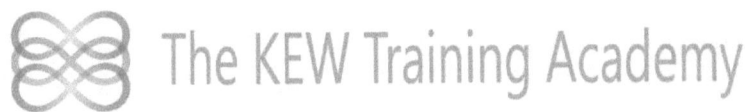

been modelling all this hypnotic language, one of them asked the other the question, "do you think we can get the same results without hypnosis?" In other words, was there a structure to what Milton did that you could use in normal waking consciousness with wide awake people?

The purpose of these hypnotic language patterns is to induce a state in some one or to change a state. Same as a parable, or a metaphor or a story.

Conversational hypnosis is a powerful form of excellence in human communication used quite naturally and effectively by successful and persuasive professionals in every field of endeavour. It can be adapted for use in many situations.

The "Milton Model": Hypnotic Language Patterns

Milton Model patterns are all about chunking up and gaining agreement. This is especially useful in business, management, coaching and relationships especially when the patterns are used outside of the conscious awareness of the listener.

Conversational Hypnosis

Here are some hypnotic sentences. Read through the list a few times, practice and then start to create some of your own.

- It's easy to discover something special deep inside.

- You may have noticed, (name), extraordinary qualities in yourself, you know they're there.

- Eventually you will learn the deeper meanings of those events.

- Some people, (add name), find it so easy to just relax, just relax and let go.

- A person can get tremendous satisfaction looking back and seeing they made it.

- People don't have to listen very closely to everything that I say, just the bits that are important for them.

- I wouldn't tell you to close your eyes and focus inwards because you can do that in your own time, in your own way.

- I wouldn't tell you to trust the process and let go until you feel you really want to go inside and find a comfortable safe place to dream.

- I'm wondering how soon you will discover how great it feels to have made that change.

- You may not know if your hands or your feet will begin to feel warmer first.

Hypnotherapy Practitioner Course - Professional Accredited Hypnotherapy Training

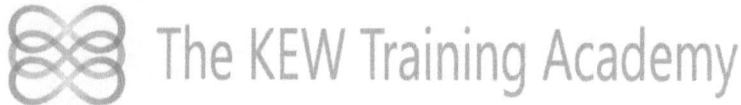

- You may not know how easily and peacefully you can just drift off into trance.

- A person could just stop (drinking, eating, smoking) quite easily and be amazed at how quickly they did it.

- If you breathe deeply and regularly you'll easily begin to go deeper.

- You may not have noticed that....(add)

- I could tell you that you'll feel very much better after this session, but I'll let you discover that for yourself.

- I could tell you that you have all the ability inside you but you probably know that already.

- A person may not know if that arm will begin to feel lighter or the other one heavier.

- When you get in touch with your inner strengths you'll find answers come quite quickly.

- When you let go of those old un-resourceful memories and let them float away, then you'll find much better, more resourceful ones will take their place.

Working with Resistant Clients

Using Ericksonian Hypnosis Language Patterns

Ericksonian language patterns are extremely effective when working with resistant or analytical clients. They are a form of indirect suggestion and can be used during normal conversation (conversational hypnosis) or throughout and during the hypnotherapy session. They allow the suggestions to go deep into the client's subconscious whilst allowing the client to still feel in control.

Here are some examples: Fill in the blanks with the suggestion that you want your clients to follow. These are called **"Embedded Commands"**.

- **Don't _____ too quickly** The suggestion here is that you're going to do it; it's just a matter of how quickly. e.g. **Don't** *go into a trance* **too quickly. Don't** *start to relax* **too quickly.**

- **I don't know exactly how _____** Not exactly, but it's going to happen.**e.g I don't know exactly how** *you're going to go into a trance*. **I don't know exactly how** *you'll find these learning's helping you the most.*

Hypnotherapy Practitioner Course - Professional Accredited Hypnotherapy Training

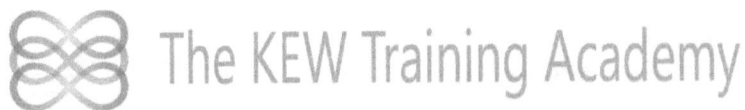

- **I wonder_____** Isn't it wonderful to wonder? Of course, when I wonder, you have to process the meaning of what I'm wondering about.

- **I wonder** if you'll *just forget that you ever had that problem*. **I wonder** what it will be like for you *to take a fresh new outlook on this situation*.

- **I wouldn't tell you to _____ because_____** I wouldn't tell you to, so you don't need to resist against it. And just to make sure, I'll give you a reason (people love reasons).e.g. **I wouldn't tell you to** relax *the muscles in your arms and legs* **because** *it's up to you how you prepare to go into trance*. **I wouldn't tell you to** *enjoy the process of going into trance* **because** *it goes without saying that you will*.

- **I'm curious to know_____**I'm not asking you, I'm just saying that I'm curious. e.g. **I'm curious to know** *how deeply you'll go into trance*.**I'm curious to know** *which resources you'll find to deal with this*.

- **What happens when you_____** I'm only asking. But to find out what happens, you have to do it.e.g. **What happens when you** *imagine yourself enjoying all the benefits of having made this change?* **What happens when** *you imagine being able to use these language patterns effortlessly?*

- **I don't know whether_____**I don't know, but you'll know, once you've considered the possibilities. e.g. **I don't know whether** *you can feel a tingling sensation in your fingers.***I don't know whether** *you've decided just how deeply you're going to embed these patterns in your language*.

- **Can you imagine_____**Can you imagine it? You have to imagine it to find out if you can or not.e.g. **Can you imagine** *going into the deepest trance you've ever experienced?* **Can you imagine** *waking up to find that this problem has just disappeared?*

- **You may already have started to notice the changes in_____ as you _____**When I say that you may have started to notice something, you check to find out if you have or not. And while you're checking, it's just so tempting to just accept what follows the "as you". e.g. **You may already have started to notice the changes in** *your physical sensations* **as you** *allow yourself to relax into a trance*. **You may already have started to notice the changes in** *your depth of trance* **as you** *focus on the feeling of going deeper*.

- **A person can_____**A person can. I'm not saying who, so you're unconscious assumes I mean you. e.g. **A person can** *relax easily*. **A person can** *get in touch with their own creativity*.

- **A person can** *find imaginative ways to use these language patterns with others*.

Hypnotherapy Practitioner Course - Professional Accredited Hypnotherapy Training

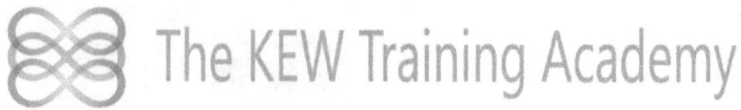

Stopping Smoking with Hypnotherapy

Successful Smoking Cessation Session

- Smoking Questionnaire – gives them time to reflect and really think about their reasons for stopping smoking

- Go through questionnaire answers with the client gathering as much information that you can to use later in your session

- 19 Deadly Poisons in Cigarettes – Is it really worth it??

- Mind Model – How Hypnotherapy Works

- Suggestibility Test – Show the power of the mind

- Do you have any questions before you stop smoking?

- Relaxation Technique – Induction

- Deepener

- Therapy Work / Script

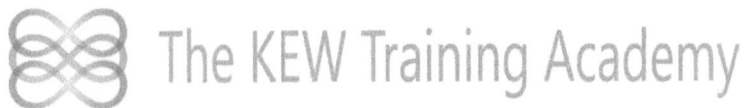
The KEW Training Academy

Smoking Questionnaire – Example 1

Name:...

Age:...

Marital Status:..

Occupation:...

Is your work stressful? No Moderately Very

Partners name:..

 Age:...

Children:.............................. Children's Names:...

Do any others in your family smoke? Yes No

How many cigarettes do you smoke in a day? ....

At what age did you start smoking? ....

Why did you re-start? Peer Pressure, Rebel against authority, To appear more adult

Other:...

What do you get from smoking? It relaxes me,It helps me to concentrate,It's an excuse for a break,It gives me a confidence boost, It's a prop.

Other:...

When do you smoke? On waking,At breakfast, With tea/coffee, After meals,Driving, On the phone,At work, In bed

Other:...

What frightens you about smoking?
....
....
What is your main motivation for stopping smoking?
....

Hypnotherapy Practitioner Course - Professional Accredited Hypnotherapy Training

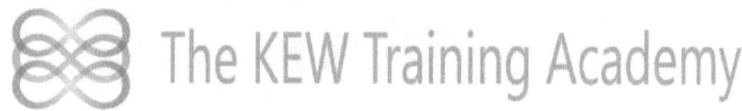

....

Do you know someone who has died from a smoking related disease?

Yes No If so who?

....

Do you know someone who is ill now? Yes No

What is important to you?

....
....

Who are you important to and why?

....
....

Has your doctor mentioned your smoking? Have you ever had any worrying symptoms? Do you have any health problems?

Heart problems High blood pressure

Yes No Yes No

Asthma

Diabetes Ulcers Other:.....................................

How long do you want to live?

....

Why?

....
....

Who is responsible for your health?

....

What will you be able to do as a non-smoker that you could not do before?

....
....

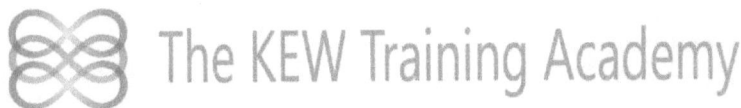

What will you do with the money that you save?

....
....

Do you really wish to commit yourself to stopping smoking?

Yes No

What is stopping you?

....

On a scale of 1 to 10, with 10 being totally determined and committed to stopping smoking, what number are you on the scale at the moment?

....

If you're not a 10 on the scale, what do you think needs to happen in order for you to be a 10 on the scale?

....

What do you need to think about cigarettes?

....

What do you need to see them as?

....

How do you need to feel about them?

....

Are you 100% committed to stopping smoking today? Yes No

Signed...

Date: ....

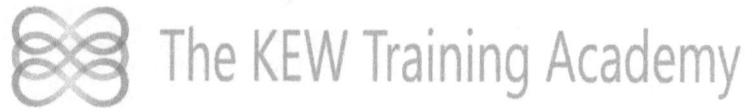

Stopping Smoking Questionnaire – Example 2

Name: ....

Age:...........................

Marital Status:.....................

Occupation:.............. ....

Is your work stressful? No Moderately Very

Partners   name: ....
Age:....................................

Children:...

Children's Names:...

(Please   circle   or   delete   where   appropriate)
How many cigarettes do you smoke a day (approximately)

1-5: 6-10: 10-15: 16-20: 20-30: 31+

Where do you smoke most of your cigarettes?

....

Are you usually in company with other smokers or alone when you smoke? Company/Alone

Do you live with anyone else who smokes?

Do any of your work colleagues smoke?

Do you smoke at work?

Have you stopped smoking before?

If yes, how long did you stop smoking for?

....

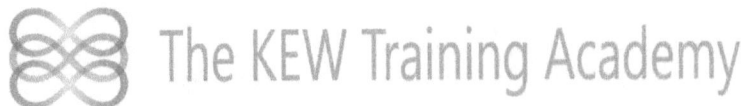

What method did you use? (Please circle)

Nicotine Patches: Chewing Gum: Hypnotherapy: Willpower: Other

....

What prompted you to start smoking again?

....

What emotions do you associate with the reason why you started smoking? i.e. guilt, comfort, punishment, contentment, stress, peer-pressure, etc.

....

Where and when do you have the first cigarette of the day

....

Do you smoke after meals? Yes/ No Do you smoke more in social situations? Yes/ No

Do you have any major stresses in your life at present? If yes, briefly describe below:

....
....

Do you suffer from breathing difficulties?

Do you suffer from colds, coughs and/or flu?

Are you health conscious?

Would you describe your health as: Excellent/ Good/ Fair/ Poor

Has any member of your family died through smoking related illnesses? Yes/ No:

What benefit does smoking have for you?

....

Why do you want to stop smoking?

....

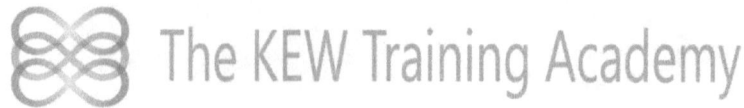
The KEW Training Academy

Identifying behaviour patterns

Thinking about the reasons or situations why and when you smoke now, please list the three which most apply to you from the following list, or substitute for your own.

- I smoke more when I Stressed
- Bored
- Driving After lovemaking
- Irritable Walking
- Angry
- Upset
- Relaxing
- Thinking To escape pressure
- After meals
- Lonely
- Talking on the telephone
- Socializing
- Nervous
- Talking
- Happy

What is important to you?

....

Who are you important to? Why?

....

How long do you want to live? Why?

....

Who is responsible for your health?

....

What will you be able to do as a non-smoker that you could not do before?

....

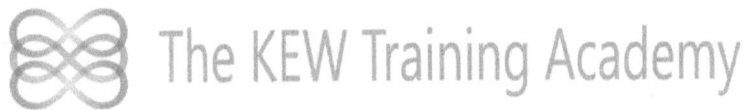

What will you do with the money that you save?

....

Think about your goal date for stopping smoking.

If you are an 'all or nothing' type of personality you may be better of stopping smoking straight away (i.e. after one session of hypnotherapy). However, if you have any stress in your life, or prefer to cut down before quitting, decide on a date and write it in the space provided.

I pledge to myself that I will stop smoking on

....

Now sign this as a commitment to yourself

....

Reasons For Smoking

Clients sometimes feel they are losing something when they become a Non Smoker. Your job is to show them that cigarettes can't give them those things. Eg confidence, this doesn't come from cigarettes, it's always been inside of them. Do this in trance where your reframes make a greater impact

Common Reason (Excuses) For Smoking

1. Confidence
2. An excuse for a break at work
3. To celebrate something
4. Relaxation
5. As an end of day ritual
6. Part of drinking something eg alcohol or coffee
7. To accompany meals
8. Part of socialising
9. To avoid boredom
10. Quiet time to think about things
11. To signal a time for them to have a private chat with
12. someone (usually a partner)
13. To concentrate on a task

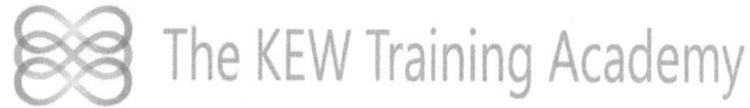

Deadly Poisons in Cigarettes

Cigarettes are one of few products which can be sold legally which can harm and even kill you over time.

Here's a list of just some of the deadly poisons in cigarettes:

Benzene (petrol additive) *A colourless cyclic hydrocarbon obtained from coal and petroleum, used as a solvent in fuel and in chemical manufacture - and contained in cigarette smoke. It is a known carcinogen and is associated with leukaemia.*

Formaldehyde (embalming fluid) *A colourless liquid, highly poisonous, used to preserve dead bodies - also found in cigarette smoke. Known to cause cancer, respiratory, skin and gastrointestinal problems.*

Ammonia (toilet cleaner) *Used as flavouring, frees nicotine from tobacco turning it into a gas, found in dry cleaning fluids.*

Acetone (nail polish remover) *Fragrant volatile liquid ketone, used as a solvent, for example, nail polish remover - found in cigarette smoke.*

Tar *Particulate matter drawn into lungs when you inhale on a lighted cigarette. Once inhaled, smoke condenses and about 70 per cent of the tar in the smoke is deposited in the smoker's lungs.*

Nicotine (insecticide/addictive drug)*One of the most addictive substances known to man, a powerful and fast-acting medical and non-medical poison. This is the chemical which causes addiction.*

Carbon Monoxide (CO) (car exhaust fumes) *An odourless, tasteless and poisonous gas, rapidly fatal in large amounts - it's the same gas that comes out of car exhausts and is the main gas in cigarette smoke, formed when the cigarette is lit. Others you may recognize are :*

Arsenic *(rat poison),* **Hydrogen Cyanide** *(gas chamber poison)*

Get Your Clients Motivated

Does Your Client really want to quit smoking? How motivated are they?

Discover the reason they want to quit. Usually it's Family and/or Health and/or Money.

Test their Motivation – look at them meaningfully and say –

"Are you absolutely sure that you really want to quit right now!?!"

There are only 3 reactions to this:

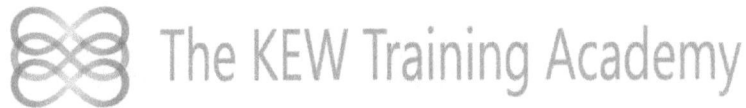
1. "YES!" – the client is ready for the main session

2. "Erm...yeah..sure" – an incongruent yes means you reframe the Client

3. "Ummmm... I don't think so" – if they say No that means you either reframe the client or do not proceed with the session.

You only want to work with clients who are enthusiastic about getting results and are 100% convinced they want to stop smoking. Otherwise you HAVE TO send them away to really think about it.

The Dickens Process – Smoking Change & Motivation, Weight Loss, Stop Smoking

Freely adapt the script to your client's needs and personality (and your style of delivery), changing wording as you see fit, to accomplish the goal. The goal here is to make the client highly suggestible for suggestions associated to the change they want to make. This is vividly accomplished by way of comparing, what they have been doing along with its outcome (i.e., the difficulties that smoking causes), and the likely outcome of making the change (i.e. better health as a non-smoker).

In the script, doing the easy thing (taking the Low Road), is associated with ultimate failure, while putting some effort into making the change is associated with ultimate success and achievement (taking the High Road).

When you take your client down the Low Road, remember to have her become aware of the people and objects associated with that low and painful road. For example, if working with a smoker, as you go down the bad road of smoking, have her look at all of the cigarette butts and ashtrays along the way, so that the emotional pain of the Low Road experience becomes associated with those items. If you are working with a substance abuser, have her look at all of the paraphernalia and drug-using friends that are all along that road. This is useful because it helps your client to break free from associating pleasure with these items and individuals. Then they can begin to associate pleasure and success with the people and things on the road on the right as you point them out.

The High Road To Success: As A Non smoker

*Today you are standing at a fork in the road of your life. You have come to a decision point. Should you continue to do what you have been doing with regard to **smoking**?*

*You think about all the problems and concerns that **smoking** brings into your life.*

(Mention some of the reasons your client told you she wants to make the change).

You think about how it has robbed you of money, energy, health, and having a sense of control over your life.

The road on the left is a slow downward road. It is easy to take the Low Road. You could just coast down it. It is the path of doing what you have been doing for so long, **by continuing to smoke**. *But, it is a path of misery. The road on the right goes upward. It will take some effort to take the High Road. But, it is the way of freedom, health and life. It is the road of being in control of your life. It is the High Road To Success!* **It is the road you have decided to take as a non-smoker.**

Look at the road on the left. It means carrying all of the problems associated with continuing to **smoke** *with you even longer than you already have. Think of how bad* **smoking** *makes you feel. Really allow yourself to feel the weight of the burden of this self- destructive behaviour. Feel your desire to be free from all of the ill effects of hurting yourself* **by smoking and taking poison into your body**.

I'm going to count from 1 to 3, and we are going to go down that low road of being out of control one more year. 1, 2, 3! There you are, after one more year of being out of control--of being miserable because you have continued to **smoke cigarettes**. *You feel the weight of the disappointment in yourself. You notice the things that litter this painful way of living-***filthy ashtrays, burns in fabrics and furniture, and the smell! You see a road littered with cigarette butts, and cartons or packs of cigarettes. You see them and they make you feel this way.** *(mention the associated paraphernalia, such as ashtrays, bottles, etc.)* **You see others that you know, who smoke, maybe it is the ones that you have smoked with, or others that you have seen huddled together outside of buildings or stuck in the smoking section of restaurants, and the sight of them makes you feel sorry for them, they are stuck on the Low Road of being a smoker.** *(If it seems appropriate to the issue, point out the people associated with the problem, the bad influences.)* *There is a mirror there and you see yourself and you ask yourself, Am I pleased with myself? Am I happy to have another year* **of smoking cigarettes**? *Do I feel better having made this decision? Do I feel healthier or worse? Do I look and feel better about myself, or not? Do I feel smarter? Feel the disappointment you have in yourself for continuing to* **smoke** *for another year!*

I'm going to count from 1 to 3 and we are going to go down to the 5 year point on this road of a **smoker** *to the year _____! 1, 2, 3! There you are after 5 more years of being on the Low Road. Bring forth all of the effects of that choice! Really allow yourself to feel the effects of that decision. You feel* **unhealthy, worried about the effects of putting tobacco poison in your mouth every day**. *You feel hopeless. Now look around you and you see all of* **those cartons and packs of cigarettes that you have bought, the dirty stinking ashtrays, the buts, the smell on your clothes and hands and face, and you hate it because it brings in all of these terrible feelings of feeling out of control, a victim of tobacco marketing.** *(Mention items associated with the problem, i.e., ashtrays, or candy wrappers, etc). Those are the things that have done this to you. So, you can't stand them anymore. Maybe you even hate the sight of them.* **You see others on the path, and they look terrible and they feel terrible.**

They are outsiders. Society is pushing them out, because they seem so ignorant or stubborn and they smell. No one wants them around their children, or to be around them socially or even at work because they smell. You may have smoked with some of these people. Are they really your friends? Do they really care about you? Again, you ask yourself, Am I pleased with myself for **smoking** for 5 more years? Do I have the right to do this to myself? Am I healthier for **smoking**? How is it affecting my life? Is my life better or worse? Do I feel smarter for **smoki**ng for an additional 5 years?

And now I count from 1 to 3 and we move down to the 10-year point on this low road of continuing to the year_____. 1, 2, 3! There you are after 10 more years of hurting yourself by **smoking**. Once again, bring forth all of the cumulative effects of that choice! Really allow yourself to feel the effects of that decision, of continuing to **smoke** for 10 more years. You feel **tired and worried about your health**. You feel more hopeless. Again, you look around you and you see all of the **things that are associated with making you feel this way, the ashtrays, the cigarette butts, the pack and cartons of tobacco poison in the form of cigarettes** (mention items associated with the problem, i.e., ashtrays, or candy wrappers, etc). *Those are the things that have done this to you. So, you can't stand them anymore. Maybe, you even hate the sight of them.* **Just looking at all that stuff associated with smoking makes you feel this way. You see the others who are on the road of being out of control with smoking. Maybe you wish you could help them. Some may be family or friends. Notice, how seeing them smoke makes you feel about cigarettes.** There is a mirror there and you look at yourself. You ask yourself, Am I pleased with myself for **smoking** for 10 more years? Is my life better or worse? Do I feel intelligent for **being a smoker** for an additional 10 years? Really feel the consequences of remaining on this low but easy road.

As I count back from 5 to 1, you come all the way back to the beginning of the fork in the road. 5, 4, 3, 2, 1. And, you feel better because none of that has to happen yet and it doesn't have to... You have decided not to let that happen to you. You have decided to take the High Road of Success on the right! You know that it will take a little more effort, but now you know in your heart and mind that it is worth it. You have decided to start taking better care of yourself! In fact you have already left the old way by coming here today! You are already taking your first steps toward freedom and success on the road on the right **as a non-smoker for good!**

Let's see how this new decision to **be free from the smoking habit** for life affects you. You think about all the good positive changes that becoming free from the self-destructive habit has brought into your life! Being free from all those problems--the feeling of really being in control and confident. You are now on the path on the right, it means success and a feeling of energy and optimism. **You have more energy. You feel more in control. You feel more self-confident, even smarter. You are free of all of the worries, costs and inconveniences that cigarettes cause.**

I'm going to count from 1 to 3, and we are going to go down that road of **being a free, non-smoker. Of** having made this **healthy** change for one year. 1, 2, 3! There you are after one year of being in control, **of being a non-smoker**. *You feel good, great! You have done it! You are a success and you never felt better and you are going to feel even better yet! There is a mirror there and you see yourself and you ask yourself, Am I pleased with myself? Am I happy to have accomplished my goal* **of being a non-smoker** *for a whole year?* **There are some new things in your life because you are more active and energetic. You are spending more and more time with friends that are on this High Road of success. You have inspired others to make this good healthy choice.** (If it seems appropriate to the problem, point out the things/items and people associated with this new way of living and being.) *Do I feel better having made this healthy decision? Do I feel smarter? Feel the pride and health that is inside of you. Was it worth it? Do you want to continue to stay on the High Road of Success?* **You have decided that this life of a non-smoker is the right life for you.**

I'm going to count from 1 to 3 and we are going to go down to the 5 year point on this road of being a success in **becoming a non- smoker** *to the year_____! 1,2,3! There you are after 5 more years of success, of reaping the rewards of making this permanent change in how you* **feel. You have found other ways to relax or take a break. Good healthy ways to take a break when you want to**. *5 years of being in control and energized! Bring forth right now all of the effects of that choice! Really allow yourself to feel the effects of that decision. You feel strong.* **This is how it feels as a non-smoker.** *Everything in your life is better for having made this permanent change. Enjoy the feeling of knowing that you have made a permanent change, knowing that you will never go back to the old way.*

And now I count from 1 to 3 and we move down to the 10-year point on this High Road of Success to the year _____. 1, 2, 3, and there you are after 10 more years of making this good and positive change in your life. Bring forth all of the effects of that smart choice! Really allow yourself to feel the effects of this decision, of continuing to be in control for 10 more years.

Smoking *is now simply something that you used to do. It was a mistake to have ever* **smoked,** *but now you are free and will remain free for the rest of your life! You look into that mirror one more time and ask yourself, Am I pleased with myself for* **kicking that old disgusting habit** *for 10 more years? Would I ever go back to that old bad habit of hurting myself by* **smoking**? *Am I glad that I have made this permanent change? A change made for good! Of course you are!*

I count back to 1 and you are back in the year _____, 5,4,3,2,1. You now have a new found level of certainty that you are ready--really ready to make this change! You are now ready to accept powerful hypnotic suggestion to help to keep you on the road on the right, the High Road of Success, **the road of a non-smoker.** *Now your subconscious mind fully accepts the suggestion that you will never* **smoke** *again. From now on you will* **always be a non-smoker, free to be happier and healthier for the rest of your life!** *This keeps you on the High Road of Success on the right.* (Repeat and add benefits that your client expects to receive from making this change. For example, *"Now that you have decided*

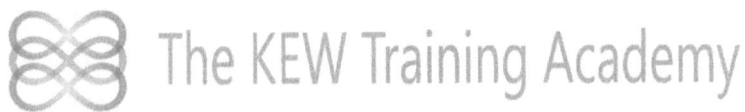

*to become a non-smoker for good, you will find **that you have improved your life in every way!**)*

The Road to Success as a Non Smoker

You are standing at a crossroad of your life. You've been travelling along this road for (number of years as a smoker), and as you see, the road continues for many miles. But now you've reached the crossroad and have the opportunity to take a different path – but you're not sure how life will be if you change course at this point in your life.

So let us continue, for a few moments more, along this old, familiar path, and see if we can see what life has in store for those who continue to smoke. Walk along the path of continuing to smoke in this way and see along your path, all the things associated with smoking. The dirty ashtrays overflowing with four smelling cigarette ends, the thick smoke that gets under your skin and in your hair and even in your lungs – making you cough and wheeze, gasping for breath along the way. Notice the smell of your clothes as you walk along the path, you feel self-conscious and try to keep your distance from non-smokers, because you're embarrassed about how your clothes and hair and skin smell so awful.

And you continue to walk along the road of continuing to smoke, seeing other smokers along   the   way   and   they   are   coughing too. You pass a hospital and remember someone in there – gasping desperately for every single breath, reaching out for a breathing apparatus, and you feel so sorry for that person because there is nothing you can do.

As you continue along the path you see yourself in years to come with children – grandchildren – babies who you aren't allowed to hold in case you breathe on them and leave that stale unpleasant smell behind. You see yourself having very little money, yet scraping it together to buy a packet of fags, then setting fire to each and every one – whilst at the same time – trying to kill yourself with poison.

You see your yellowed fingers with nicotine stains and that nasty, nauseous smell. Your skin feels tight and dirty and you're coughing and wheezing all the time. That tickly cough just won't go away.

You see yourself as an outcast – no-one wants to know you. At work you have to go outside to smoke. In company you feel alienated as you notice those few friends you have, inching away from you as they hold their nose – trying not to inhale that stench.

You see burn marks in your home and walls that are stained yellow from the smoke. Furnishings too, have that stale, unpleasant smell. And as you continue to the end of this road, see yourself in hospital, like that friend before you, frightened and fighting for your breath.

And all these things that you see, along the way, are associated in your mind, and rightly so, with smoking.

Now let us leave that scene for now, because none of that has happened, and because it's not going to happen. You have reached the crossroad of your life. By coming here today, you have already decided that it's time to make that change. You've seen the things that could happen if you continued on that road, now let us see what life will really be like for you. Take the new road now – the road to success at being a non-smoker. Come with me for a moment and let us see what's on this new road of success.

The first thing that you notice is how clean the air is here. Everything is crystal clear, and you breathe in pure air, you can actually breathe in that fresh, crystal clean, pure air. Just see how good it makes you feel, as you walk along the road. The air fills your being with renewed energy and vitality and already, after just a short time of being a non-smoker, you find that you're feeling better and healthier than ever before.

You notice how you're breathing is so much easier than before. Your chest feels comfortable and your throat nice and clear. Your skin feels better and your fingers are a healthy colour.

You notice too, how clean and fresh you smell, your clothes, your skin, your hair – a lovely fresh, clean smell, a delicate smell, that faint perfume by which people now recognise you. Notice the people along the road to success, they all admire you because you said you could be a non-smoker, and you did it. You kept your word, you made a conscious decision to quit the habit of smoking once and for all, and you did it. People you love, like to be close to you, because you smell clean and nice and fresh.

And instead of a hospital you a place of entertainment, a sports complex or a gymnasium, or some other place where you enjoy being, and keeping fit and healthy, with friends or people you love – with others that you have inspired to also make that healthy choice, to become and remain, non-smokers, for the rest of their lives.

You have more confidence in yourself because you rely on yourself, instead of props or addictions – you are your own person – self- confident, self-assured – you have wonderful feelings of achievement and attainment and wellbeing, now that you're a non- smoker.

You see your home - a beautiful place to be, it is clean and fresh and well maintained, no sign of smoke or tar or nicotine or cigarettes at all. Just a beautiful, peaceful place to be. And you really enjoy being here. You love the feeling of being a non- smoker, it's such a wonderful feeling for you. And every day you are more and more determined to remain a non-smoker. Every day you are more and more motivated to remain a non-smoker. Every day you feel better and healthier and fitter, you have more energy and more vitality, you feel really good about yourself.

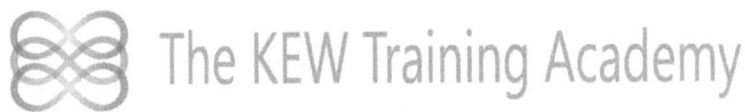

As you travel along the road to success of being a non-smoker I wonder if you can see yourself – or sense, or feel yourself, quite a long way past that crossroad of your life. Know that you're at a future date, several months from now, having succeeded at becoming a non-smoker and feeling really proud of yourself.

It's a lovely road now, new plants are springing up on either side of the road – opportunities arising for you, confidence increasing because you feel so much better about yourself, now that you're a non-smoker.

See yourself with all the money you've saved – money you would otherwise have spent on smoking – purchasing something special, perhaps a new outfit or something for your home – perhaps even putting the deposit on a holiday – it doesn't matter what, so long as it's something special for you – because you are special – you deserve to treat yourself, you deserve to feel proud of

yourself. You are a wonderful, worthwhile human being and you proved that you meant what you said, when you stopped smoking.

At this point in the road, in your future, as a non-smoker, I wonder if you can see yourself in a situation where, in the past you might have smoked.

Imagine that your so called friend is there. A friend who smokes a lot. And this friend is offering a cigarette to you. See her (him) taking out a packet of cigarettes and carefully and slowly unwrapping the cellophane from it. Then opening the packet and pulling out halfway, a cigarette to offer you.

And suddenly you realize that this friend is not a 'true' friend. No true friend would try to tempt you in this way. And that makes you feel even more determined to remain a non-smoker.

Hear yourself say 'No'. You say 'No' to cigarettes, and you mean No. Your mind and body reject cigarettes. Cigarettes are like a poison to your system. You do not want them, you do not need them, you do not have them.

And when you say 'No' to cigarettes, an amazing thing happens. You feel a wonderful feeling flowing into your being. Filling your very existence with pride and confidence and that sense of achievement again. You feel wonderful. So you say 'No' to cigarettes, and you mean No. You say No, No, No. No to cigarettes, because you're a non-smoker and that's the way you prefer to be.

Every day you feel better and healthier and happier, you have more confidence and more vitality and you feel really, really good, because you are a non-smoker now. You are a non-smoker and that's the way you really do prefer to be. Every day these suggestions will grow stronger and stronger. Every day you become more determined and more motivated to remain a non- smoker, every day you feel better and happier and healthier and fitter than ever before. You are a non-smoker now. You are a non- smoker and you prefer to be a non-smoker. And every day these suggestions grow stronger and stronger, they become more and more profound, more and more powerful and more and more important to you. In a moment I'm going to count up to five and at the count of five you will be wide, wide, wide awake. You'll have beautiful feelings flowing through your body, calm and peaceful thoughts flowing through your mind. And these wonderful thoughts and feelings will remain with you. They will remain and stay with you.

Guilt Trip

This technique is very effective when used towards the end of a session. This approach can be used for so many negative behaviours. Simply substituting the word "smoking" with "over eating", for example, will do the trick.

As you take a deep breath now...I would like your subconscious mind to show you a room...a familiar room perhaps...gathered here are all those people who are special to you....who love and care for you and whom you love and care for. They have all come here today....because you have something to explain to them all...Your doctor has warned you that you must quit smoking because the next aneurysm/heart attack will more than probably prove fatal...You will die an early death because you refuse to take responsibility for your own life and your own health....For the sake of a noxious habit you are prepared to risk all....In fact you have made a choice....a choice to die an early death leaving behind all of these people who so much wish for you to give up that dreadful habit....Now I want you to explain to all here why you choose to continue to smoke....to risk with every cigarette that life that is so precious....not just to you...but to those here who rely on you to be there for them....Go ahead and tell them why a cigarette means so much more to you than the love and care that they give to you....much more than the life that is so precious....Tell them now the awful truth...and watch their faces....the dismay....the horror....the disgust....the feelings of helplessness....anger....grief....and how do you feel now?

(Await response and then continue with session)

Amnesia

It can be useful for the client not to retain memory of session content if rationalisation could prove detrimental to what has been achieved subconsciously.

As you drift and dream....continuing to relax in that special way....breathing easily....quietly....relaxing deeper and deeper with every gentle breath....i wonder if you can recall how much you have concerned yourself with those thoughts...those fleeting memories of events...ideas that drift in and out...the subconscious mind can work so hard when it relaxes too....and then you can become so aware of how difficult it can be to recall what I was telling you five minutes ago....and then what if you could remember what I said seven and a half minutes ago....what you were thinking....just a minute ago....or even four minutes ago....it really can seem to be just too much effort to make....to try to

Hypnotherapy Practitioner Course - Professional Accredited Hypnotherapy Training

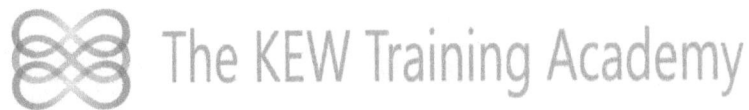

remember....not worth the bother....so much easier to just allow that relaxation....that comfortable time to continue....with a knowing that you really have no need at all to concern yourself at all.....

I wonder if you are aware, that good co-operative hypnotic subjects are so easy to spot as they close their eyes just as you are doing now? It can be such a relaxing experience ....

Confusion Technique to Facilitate Amnesia

And now that you have had the opportunity to discover new possibilities....while you can learn from past experiences....your conscious mind can begin to wonder how it will know which things to remember....and which things only your subconscious need now...and then you can remember to forget....or you may choose to forget to remember....Your memory of forgetting forgets what it has forgotten...but you can only forget what you have forgotten when you realise it's too difficult to remember anyway.....and then when you can forget all the confusion...and relax even more deeply than before....

Instilling Confidence in Clients

There are several ways that you can help clients who present with low self-esteem and lack of self-confidence.

In most, if not all cases, low self-esteem and lack of confidence stem from earlier issues in a client's life. A few examples are:

1. Lack of support and encouragement from parents, grand- parents, teachers and/or other care-givers:

2. Being bullied at school or feeling alienated, excluded or different from other children;

3. Sibling rivalry;

4. Physical, mental, emotional or sexual abuse;

Of course, every client is different and their whole life experiences depend upon their personal circumstances and how they feel that they fit into the world.

An understanding and empathic therapist will help a client to understand the psycho-dynamics of how and why they feel lacking or inferior and empower the client with a new and healthier set of perspectives.

My first step when dealing with this issue is to explore my client's background; the position in the family, who they felt closest to, how supported they felt, if parents divorced, which one did they live with? Was there any history of family violence? How did they interact with teachers and peers at school or later with their work colleagues?

Each set of questions will depend upon the answers given to previous questions; my main concern is to understand where my client is coming from.

Then I will establish, in what circumstances does my client feel uncomfortable? Some people are fine with family and close friends but not with a group or with people they believe to be superior to them. Every little piece of information that you gather is important in order to see the whole picture.

If a client has absolutely no idea why they feel this way then I would suggest regression to cause, but not usually in the first session, unless they've been before for some other issue and I know that they are a good hypnotic subject.

It's also important to ascertain how your client will know that they are feeling more confident in the future - what single thing will tell them that they are progressing?

So, the first session will be a gathering of information, followed by a gentle hypnotic induction and suggestions of calm, relaxation and confidence, together with a post-hypnotic suggestion (usually an anchor/key word to trigger off positive feelings when necessary).

Mental rehearsal is used to allow the subject to see themselves behaving in a more positive way. Mental rehearsal lies down neural-pathways in the brain which allows a client to feel that they have already experienced this positive feeling or situation, making it easier for when they physically experience it (in a non-hypnosis situation).

Good feelings can be anchored by amplifying them in hypnosis and having a client press together a thumb and finger and taking some deep breaths, perhaps also conjuring up a key word or phrase, so that whenever they need to feel this way again, they just need to use their anchor/trigger.

Clients may be asked to form a circle around themselves and draw symbols inside to represent any positive thoughts or feelings about themselves. Alternatively they may write things they dislike about themselves on a blackboard and wipe them all away and out out their life, replacing them with positive qualities.

Use your imagination when working with clients - work with visualizations about things that they are interested in. For example, someone interested in computers might see themselves going into the start program on Windows and selecting Add or Remove Programs; they can delete any unwanted ones and add new ones.

In a similar way they could visualize themselves on a pebbly beach - selecting pebbles that symbolize some old negative thought or feeling or experience from the past and on

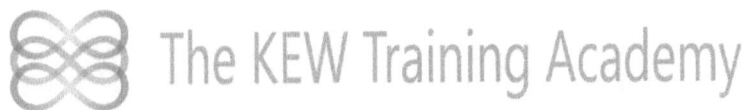

identifying it, have them throw it into the sea and watch the waves carry it away. This could also be accomplished with leaves falling into a garden, sweeping them all into a pile and having a bonfire - or a funeral for those old negative feelings.

Generating a more desired pattern of behaviour can be done by having the client think of someone whose qualities they would like to adopt; this is also known as modelling - they can see the other person behaving and acting the way that they would like to — then step into that person and experience themselves feeling and acting in exactly the same way, or a way more suited to them.

If your client's problem stem from an abusive childhood then perhaps it's time for them to let go of the past. Forgiveness is a great healer. You can emphasize that they past has passed and the present is now and the most important thing is concentrating on enjoying the present and looking forward to building a happier future.

The main thing is to be creative, use the scripts only as a framework and change and adapt them to make them your own; actively listen to your client - not only to what they are saying but listen to the unspoken messages too - they will often contain far more information that is relevant to your treatment plan.

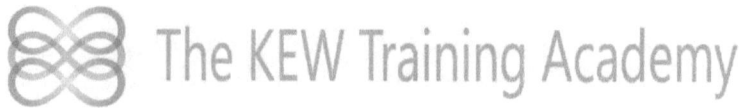

Hypnotherapy Confidence Questionnaire

Name: ....

Age:............................

Marital Status:......................

Occupation: ....

Is your life stressful? No Moderately Very

If so, in what ways is it stressful?

....

Partners name: ....

Age:....................................

Children:................................

Children's Names: ....

What is your main outcome for the session?

....

Why haven't you been able to achieve this so far?

....

What has to happen for you to feel confident and that you are good enough?

....

Was there a time in the past when you were confident , if so when?

....

What positive things have you achieved in your life time so far?

....

What are your best qualities?

....

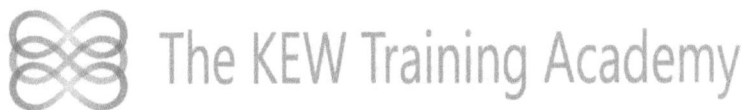
The KEW Training Academy

How do others see you?

....

Describe yourself in 3 words?

....

What are your 3 main goals?

....

What is important to you in life

....

Who are you important to and why?

....

Do you suffer from depression? Yes No

Are you on any medication ? Yes No

What will you be able to do as a more confident person that you could not do before

....

....
Would you like to be an inspiration to others? Yes No

What is stopping you then?

....
....

Are you 100% committed to making changes today and stepping out of your comfort zone?

Yes No

Signed...Date:...

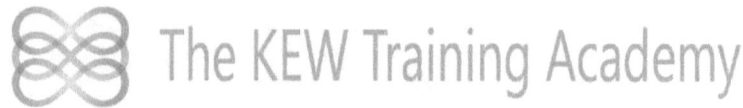

Anchoring Confidence

Begin with an induction and deepener.

Note: Ascertain whether subject is right or left handed. If left handed please reverse the mention of handedness in this script

As you drift....so comfortable now....just concentrating on the sound of my voice......you can really begin to start experiencing that feeling of knowing that you really can start to take control....using your own ability to relax....to let go....moving inwards now into your own subconscious mind where nothing at all concerns you as you distance yourself from the world around you.... Feeling totally relaxed, calm and secure.

As you continue to relax...all is tranquil and at peace...recognising now the signs of that deep hypnotic trance.... Arms feeling heavy and totally relaxed....legs feeling relaxed....your entire body seems to float now in time and space... floating peacefully as you drift and leave everything behind.....without a care in the world.

So many people come here to ask me to help them to be more confident and to make positive changes in their lives....and I tell them....that those changes are there to be made.... and that all that is needed here is a recognition of the abilities and capabilities that are already yours....to recognise that you really do have the confidence and the determination to do anything that you want to in life.

It's just like setting out on a journey....knowing that you have prepared well....everything is packed....passports and tickets are in a safe place....all arrangements have been made....knowing that **you can** and **you will** complete your journey easily and without effort....you have all the ability, capability and confidence to do what you want....to make new and good things happen....to help others....you tell yourself now**...”I can”**....**”I will”** and you feel at ease...comfortable within yourself.

And as you relax even more deeply now, you become aware of your own positive resources and you allow your subconscious mind to provide you with a memory of a time when you felt really good about yourself – perhaps you had accomplished something you were proud of or maybe you were being complimented for your effort – the content of the memory is not important – what is important now is the feeling that this memory generates within you.

And when you have that recaptured that particular memory I want you to expand upon it – see the situation that you are in, who is with you – what you are doing and where you are – then fill in the details – the time of year, spring, summer, autumn or winter – the time of the day, morning, afternoon or evening – what you are wearing and feeling and seeing and touching – if anything – hear what it is that is being said – if anything is said – or any other sounds – or smells – and now focus on the feelings, and I want you to really remember how it felt inside – those good, positive feelings, strong feelings – confident and self-assured feelings – and you can allow those good feelings to grow stronger and more positive whilst you take in a really long, deep breath in through your nose and press together the thumb and the middle finger of the right hand, whilst your subconscious mind memorizes those wonderful, confident, positive feelings.

Because in future, whenever you take in a really long, deep breath through your nose and press together the thumb and the middle finger of the right hand, as you are doing right now, you are going to feel those good, strong, confident feelings – and you can feel these good feelings anytime you wish, anywhere, in any situation. Because these good, strong, confident feelings are becoming more and more a part of you and you are becoming that stronger, more confident person. And remember, anytime you want to feel even more confident, all you need to do is to breathe in that really long, deep breath through your nose and press together the thumb and the middle finger of the right hand, and you will feel those good, strong, confident feelings filling your being. You can feel wonderful. Calmer, more relaxed, and much more confident than ever before. You know what it's like to feel those good, strong, confident feelings – and you can really enjoy remembering and re-experiencing those feelings which are becoming more and more a permanent part of you.

Now visualize yourself in a situation where you would previously have felt apprehensive or nervous in some way. Remember a particular event if you wish, in which you had wished that you'd dealt with differently. And I'd like you to walk into that situation again, relive it right now, here in the safety of hypnosis, but this time, you are taking with you the tools that you need to feel better inside – and you have those tools right here at your fingertips and right here in the air that your breathe. So take that long, slow, deep breath now – in through your nose, and press together once more the thumb and the middle finger on that right hand – and you will once again feel those strong, confident positive feelings flowing back into your awareness – filling your entire being with the strength to successfully deal with this situation.

And see or feel or sense yourself now, effectively interacting in a very confident way, a very self-assured way, a very assertive way. And as you watch yourself in this way, feel the pride that you have for yourself – the sense of calm assurance – the quiet inner calm. And every day you feel more positive about yourself because you know now that you really are achieving your fullest potential. You believe in yourself, and because you believe in yourself, other people believe in you, too.

You begin to recognize all the good things that you have done in your life and you now feel good about yourself. You are your own best friend. You have a relaxed attitude towards yourself and other people and this makes you feel more confident with those that you meet. You are kind to other people and you are kind to yourself. You give people the benefit of the doubt and build up positive relationships with those around you, because you feel at ease with people and you are confident in all situations. You always approach situations with this short phrase: "I CAN DO IT" – you tell yourself that there is nothing that is physically possible that you cannot do – you can do ANYTHING that you set your mind to – because you believe in yourself – you believe in yourself and other people believe in you.

You walk with a graceful air of inner confidence and self-assurance – because you are your own best friend. You have all the confidence that you need, to deal effectively with any situation that may arise.

And just remember that, whenever you want to feel more confident and at ease, or simply to draw into your awareness those wonderfully strong, confident, positive feelings, all you need to do is to take that long, slow, deep breath, really breathe all the air into your lungs, and as you exhale, remember to squeeze together the thumb and middle finger of that right hand. Because this is the hand that you depend upon (if subject is right handed), this is your confidence hand , and those wonderful, strong, positive feelings flow right back into your awareness.

You can use this technique whenever a situation arises when you want to draw into yourself those confident feelings, and the more often you practice this technique the stronger it becomes and the more confident you feel. You feel wonderful.

Now in a moment or two I will count up to five, and at the count of five you will be wide, wide, wide awake. You'll have beautiful feelings flowing through your body, calm and peaceful thoughts flowing through your mind. And these wonderful calm and peaceful thoughts and feelings will remain with you. They will remain and they will stay with you. So get ready now as I count up to five. And come all the way back at the count of five.

1.2.3.4.5

Circle of Confidence

Before starting, find out your client's favourite place and some of the best times in their life.

Begin with your favourite induction and deepener.

You're now standing in a large and beautiful room - over there is a door and in a moment I'm going to ask you to walk over to the door and push it open - and when you do you'll find yourself in your favourite place (state name of place) and you'll be very happy to be back here.

When you're ready - walk over to the door - push the door open - push - and the door opens easily for you - now walk through - closing the door gently behind you - and look around you - you are back here in (name) and it looks exactly the same as did when you came here last - it's a wonderful, sunshiny day and there's a clear blue sky and you feel so happy to be back here.

(Describe a few details about your client's favourite place - ensuring they are relevant - e.g. if it's a city you can describe the magnificent architecture and the wonderful atmosphere - if it's a beach then describe the sea, sand, palm trees, etc).

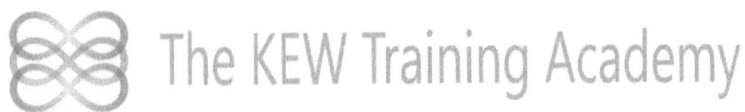

This is your perfect place - your paradise - and I want you to know that you can come back here anytime you want to - any time you want - all with the power of your wonderful subconscious mind. All you need to do is relax - and take three deep breaths - hold each one for the mental count of three - and as you breathe the air from your mouth - just think in your mind the words 'calm and relaxed' and you will instantly feel much calmer and much more relaxed - and more confident too.

Now - in your perfect place - I want you to create a circle around you - and you are standing or sitting here - in the centre of your circle - this is your circle your circle of excellence - your circle of confidence - your perfect circle.

And as you sit or stand in the centre of your circle - I want you think about all the best times in your life - all the times when you felt so good (name the instances he/she has already given and describe them as well as you can).

There may be other good times that are springing to mind - bring them here with you in your circle - perhaps a favourite holiday or times when you were complimented or had just done something good and it gave you a special feeling of pride.

And as you remember these good times - I want you to experience the good feelings again that were associated with each of these times - feelings of pride, feelings of confidence - wonderful feelings - positive feelings.

I'd like you to now create symbols for each of these feelings and events - and put those symbols into your circle - perhaps you can imagine writing them on the ground or in the sand (wherever applicable) - or maybe they're floating around you - making you feel really happy - as though you are floating on air yourself - and I'm going to be quiet for a few moments to allow you to create these symbols and feel those good feelings again - and put them all into your circle of excellence - your perfect circle - your circle of confidence.

I'll be quiet now - and when you next hear my voice you won't be startled or alarmed.

(Pause for two minutes)

Now - bring your attention back to my voice - because I want you to know and to understand that you can experience these good feelings again - whenever you want to - whenever you need to - all with the power of your own wonderful subconscious mind.

All you need to do is relax - and let go of tension - take those three deep breaths - hold each one for the mental count of three - and as you breathe out - think those words in your mind - calm and relaxed - and as you think those words in your mind = you find that you do become much more calm - and more relaxed – and much more confident too - and when you've said the words ' calm and relax' three times - I'd like you to think in your mind - my circle - just those two little words will instantly fill you with feelings of confidence and all the

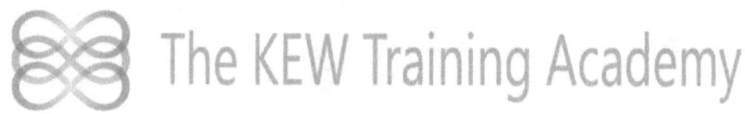
The KEW Training Academy

wonderful feelings and thoughts associated with your circle will be back in your awareness - even more powerful that they are right now.

The words - my circle - are your post hypnotic conditioned response - and when you're relaxing - in your own special time - you can go back into your circle - and you may find new things to add to it - there will be other memories springing to mind - and new experiences resulting from your newly found confidence - and you can add them to your circle of confidence - this will help to make it even stronger and more powerful for you.

And what you put into your circle - you can take out - you can take those confident feelings wherever you go - whenever you need them. Imagine yourself in a situation which previously make you feel unsure - see yourself now doing or saying or whatever it is you - with wonderful feelings of confidence - calm and happiness.

Now in a moment I'm going to count from one to five and at the count of five you'll be wide awake - feeling wonderful - and these good feelings will remain with you - they will remain and stay with you - growing stronger and stronger day by day.

So get ready now and I'll count to five and come all the way back at the count of five.... 12345...

Confidence Building

As you drift....so comfortable now....just concentrating on the sound of my voice......you can really begin to start experiencing that feeling of knowing that you really can start to take control....using your own ability to relax....to let go....moving inwards now into your own subconscious mind where nothing at all concerns you as you distance yourself from the world around you.... Feeling totally relaxed, calm and secure.

As you continue to relax...all is tranquil and at peace...recognising now the signs of that deep hypnotic trance.... Arms feeling heavy and totally relaxed....legs feeling relaxed....your entire body seems to float now in time and space... floating peacefully as you drift and leave everything behind.....without a care in the world.

So many people come here to ask me to help them to be more confident and to make positive changes in their lives....and I tell them....that those changes are there to be made.... and that all that is needed here is a recognition of the abilities and capabilities that are already yours....to recognise that you really do have the confidence and the determination to do anything that you want to in life.

It's just like setting out on a journey....knowing that you have prepared well....everything is packed....passports and tickets are in a safe place....all arrangements have been made....knowing that **you can** and **you will** complete your journey easily and without effort....you have all the ability, capability and confidence to do what you want....to make

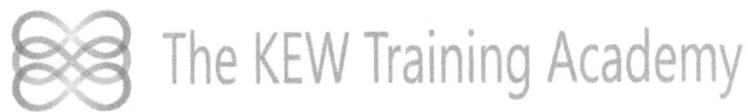

new and good things happen....to run a successful business helping others....you tell yourself now..."**I can**"...."**I will**" and you feel at ease...comfortable within yourself.

What has happened in the past has happened....from these events you have learnt so much....experiences that have helped you to grow into the strong determined person that you are today....you have overcome so much and achieved greatness that many others could never dream of doing...so you can now relax...and you can let go of all negative feelings and emotions...turning things around now and seeing the positive in everything. People from the past no longer have any influence on your life and your future... only you can determine your destiny... you are such an inspiration to others already, although you may not even realise it, and it's now time to let go of the past completely.....knowing that it served you up until a point...but you are now ready to move on to a whole new chapter of your life.... To achieve great things....from now on for you the glass is always half full.... as you refuse to accept than anybody would be thinking bad of you....negative thoughts and emotions have no place at all in your life now....they hold you back...they prevent you from being the person that you wish to be.... and that you really can be.

With every day you have learned more through experience...the best and the most effective way of learning that can be...you are the product of all your experiences...and all of those experiences that occurred way back then have only helped you to become the strong, determined woman that you are becoming today. Repeat the words in your mind "I can", I will...these words becoming embedded in your subconscious mind with immediate and lasting effect....Repeat the words three times within yourself...I can....I will....I am the equal of every person....and each day in every way...I am getting better and better.

As you now look back... on any bad memories from the past of people or events.... that have been holding you back or ....have made you lack confidence in yourself...you now begin to see things differently....you now take pride in yourself and recognise that you can be selective with any memories that you wish to keep....to place value upon...and if any memory has not been serving you with positivity...you now chose to reject those memories....to simply let them go...imagine filling up a large black bin bag with all those old negative images and memories....any hurtful words... events...anything that has been holding you back...empty them all into that bin bag now until they are all out of your head...you no longer have any need for them....and when you are done tie the bag up with a large piece of string....then I want you to take that bag to a large cliff...whenever you are ready pick up that bag and see yourself going to a large cliff and with one almighty push, throw that bag and all that old negativity over that cliff and say goodbye forever to anything or anybody holding you back. Feel a huge sense of relief....like a weight has been lifted off your shoulders and a new life has begun. This is the beginning of a bright, successful, beautiful future for you.

And as my voice drifts with you... You now look to the future in a way that tells you that things will go well.....that you will succeed.....that you are special...attractive......intelligent and capable and in this way you programme yourself to succeed and you will succeed. You now look to the future and see only good things and good people happening to you as you move forward to grasp opportunities.......clearly.....intensely....aware that all your worthwhile goals are attainable.

From now on if you ever feel any sense of self-doubt in your mind you will take 3 deep breaths and repeat to yourself "I can"..."I will" ....3 times... remembering all of the positive things that you have done in your life so far ....and all of the obstacles that you have managed to overcome...making you the positive strong woman that you are today...admired by many...an inspiration to others...and a lovely caring human being.

You have all the confidence you need within you......all the capabilities and capacities to be that person that you want to be.... Special and exciting......you and you alone have your best interests at heart..... You impress and amaze all with your clarity of thought and expression of new ideas and input to every situation......once the bystander....now at the forefront.....establishing yourself as that interesting positive person that you are.....You can now be aware that you are the equal of all.......relaxed and comfortable in every situation.....you are realising now with greater clarity each and every day.....that you can unlearn that feeling of fear and lack of confidence....You now take a deep breath........Relax yourself from head to toe....and take the image into your mind of you.....happy and secure.......confident and self-assured.....as you tell yourself.....I can....I will....This comfortable pleasant image soothes your mind, and all fear and all self-doubt leaves you completely.

You unlearn fear by being positive and realising that the only thing that can hurt you....is the fear itself......No longer do you accept fear or negativity....You banish in their entirety all unwanted inappropriate thoughts and symptoms....allowing only good thoughts and positive feelings to grow and become part of your special personality.....You do this easily because you are in control.....It will become easier and easier for you to do this as you take control.....and you will take control... won't you....

(Await response)

As you go deeper now....in control.....just listening to the sound of my voice.......your subconscious mind shows you yourself at a time.....in the past.......when you felt really confident......a time when you felt really good.....when you were the centre of attention....loved and admired.....being congratulated by those around you as you receive an award for achievement.....or realised a long standing ambition. It doesn't matter where it was or when it was.....just as long as you felt really good about yourself and about your achievement.....Think of your finest hour....and get that image into your mind as you were at that time at that place.....You see yourself right now as the centre of attention....with all others cheering you......congratulating you.....Now hold that feeling....allow that feeling to be something that expands.....Now see that special feeling as a pulsating white light....warm and comfortable.....powerful....and allow that white to expand and grow so that it encompasses you.....so that you are completely contained with a brilliant cocoon of pulsating white light......feel that warm and comfortable feeling.....confident and admiring thoughts about you and your special qualities and capabilities....Feel it growing....Expanding....filling your very being with its power and positive influence......And now... allow that white light to be absorbed into your body....as you absorb completely and permanently to your highest benefit all of those good and capable qualities that ensure that from this moment forward....you are the confident and self- assured person that you want to be.....that you are....right now.

Each and everything you do.....you do better than you ever have done before.....You approach each new task and situation with complete ease and of mind knowing that you are.....relaxed and in a perfect frame of mind....calm.....relaxed and confident......Every day your confidence grows....which means that tomorrow your confidence grows and the day after it grows stronger than before.......and as you practice being more and more confident.....so your confidence grows and becomes stronger as more and more......your feelings of self-worth become strong and powerful......Each day...with each new situation.....whenever you need to....you take control......calm your mind.....disregard troubles and you are calm......relaxed.....poised......competent......and confident.....you are your own person.....is that not so?

(wait for response and then bring client back from trance state)

Now I'm going to count you back from 10 – 1.

Hypnotherapy Script for Confidence – The Garden of Your Life

I want you to imagine, that you are standing in a beautiful garden... a garden which symbolizes your life – the garden of your life. And you are standing there, in the garden of your life, looking around at the trees and the flowers and the grass, in the garden of your life. Just nod your head to indicate to me when you are here, in this garden. Good.

Feel the warmth of the autumn sun shining down on you – the soft gentle breeze and the perfume of your favourite flowers. Notice any shrubs or bushes or other plants – perhaps an ivy-covered archway or one covered in jasmine. Perhaps you can hear the birds up there in the trees, whistling their tune to each other. Imagine it – experience it now – notice the gate over there leading out of your garden to the street beyond.

You can be happy here in the garden of your life. But first I want you to look around and notice here and there, the dried up leaves that are scattered around on the floor of your garden. Some of those leaves are yellow and some are red – in some places the leaves cover the ground almost like a thick carpet, other areas are more sparse. Now those dried up, crumpled leaves are symbolic of all the hurts and frustrations from your life.

Those crumpled, dried up leaves symbolize all the negative conditions from your past and from your present, they represent uncomfortable feelings, feelings of inadequacy, not being good enough, feelings of inferiority or embarrassment – those leaves represent all rebuttals, all refusals, all resentments, all negative statements about yourself, whether made yourself, for yourself, or by others and directed at you. All those negative statements that have been made to you at any time in your life, are all here in the garden of your life.

Now look over there – and see a rake, its long, wooden handle, the rake is propped up and I want you to take that rake and gather together all those dried and crumpled old leaves into a heap, ready to set fire to them.

And you could give names to some of those dried and crumpled old leaves. Some of the names might represent disagreeable people or events in your life, some may represent subconscious wishes for failure, there may be dislikes for some people in your life, procrastination or past negative conditioning, some may represent laziness or apathy, lack of communication or any spite or hatred or hurt that is held by you for anyone or held by anyone for you.

All these negative feelings are scattered on the ground, as you rake them into one big pile, ready for the fire. And whatever those leaves symbolize to you, we are going to 'burn them out of your life, forever'.

So when the pile is ready, I want you to set fire to those leaves, just enjoy the destruction of all those negativities. And as you do, enjoy the feeling of freedom, the feeling of being rid of all those negative influences.

And as you watch the flames leap up into the air, you feel all those negative influences from the past leaving you – totally and completely being burnt out of your life. It's as though all those negative influences from the past are going up in smoke and if you look up there you'll see that thick black smoke going higher and higher, the tail end of the smoke becoming thinner until it disperses and leaves your life forever.

And suddenly you are free. You are free from all past negative influences, all self-defeating believes, all those things that held you back in life – you are free now to progress, to advance, to achieve whatever goals you set out for yourself. You are free, and it's a wonderful feeling to be free. You feel much more confident, much more self-assured, much more comfortable with yourself.

All past negative influences have departed from your existence and it's as though you can really begin to live again – to make a fresh start, a healthy, positive start, and continuing to live a fulfilling life doing, not only the things that you have to do every day, but also the confidence to do what you really want to you.

And I want you to experience now, a beautiful violet stream of light, pouring down from the blue sky like a laser beam, in through the crown of your head. And the violet light symbolises purity of thought, because now you experience only positive thoughts and feelings, as far as is humanly possible. Feel the light entering the brain and streaming down

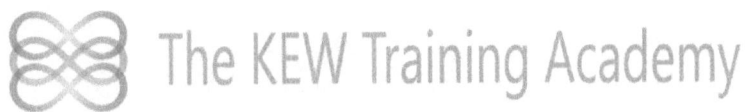
into the spinal column and out through every nerve, every cell, every fibre, every consciousness of your being. And the purity of thought and feeling touches every nerve and cell and consciousness of your being – filling you with a new healthy energy, a strong and positive energy – and you feel yourself filled with a loving acceptance of the wonderful human being that you are.

And as you accept the wonderful person that you are, you find that you begin to feel differently about yourself. You feel so much calmer, deep inside – so much more relaxed – so much more confident – and every cell in your body is bathed in love and acceptance – in a beautiful violet light – and your feelings are changing on a cellular level, even altering the chemistry of your body in a positive way.

Now Autumn and Winter have passed and it is now a warm spring sunshiny day. Out of the garden of your life, you have swept away all those negative thoughts and beliefs that you once held about yourself. Now according to the laws of nature we have to replenish what we take away, and I want you to see yourself now with a handful of special seeds.

There is an area of your garden where you instinctively know that these seeds are needed to grow. The soil is already rich and fertile and ready to take those seeds. So very carefully I want you to tenderly plant those seeds in your garden, with loving care. And sprinkle over the seeds with the soft fine earth. Shower the earth lightly to make it moist and then leave the rest to nature.

And as time goes by your seeds will grow and grow and grow. Even whilst they are growing under the earth, you won't see the shoots until they begin to peep out of the soil – but you will know that those little seeds have germinated and are sprouting up – you will know because your feelings will tell you so. You always listen carefully now to your feelings, to your inner self, that wonderful, calm and wise and confident self. Feeling that inner acceptance, loving yourself and who you are in a calm and peaceful sort of way.

When you're ready I'm going to ask you to count yourself up from one to five. At five you'll be ready to open your eyes and will feel wide awake, but even as you're rousing yourself to become aware to the external world, you know deep inside you that those seeds are already beginning to grow.

Count up when you're ready, and then open your eyes.

TimeLine

Exercise to Release Negative Emotions

1: Identify a negative attitude or a feeling you have that is holding you back. An attitude which is preventing you from fulfilling your potential, or achieving a goal, ambition, dream, living the life you deserve. Possibly an attitude which is sabotaging your relationships, stopping you from changing jobs, setting up a business. i.e. you not good enough, you're never going to succeed, you can't find a partner, you're never going to be happy or a story from your past you keep recycling which is not productive.

2a: On a piece of paper or card board write down some significant events that have happened in your past, positive and negative. (i.e. first time you fell off a bike, being told off by a parent, getting your driver's licence, graduating, your first kiss, breaking up with a partner, a bad holiday, good holiday).

2b: Now write done some of the things you're looking forward in the future. (i.e. travelling the world, writing a book, meeting someone, new job, exciting venture, getting into great shape, meeting exciting people).

2c: Now close your eyes relax and imagine a line that represents your positive future, placing all the exciting things you're looking forward to on a line that represents time.

2d: Now with your eyes closed imagine the here and now-the present.

2e: With your eyes closed imagine those past events you wrote down, as you imagine all your past events imagine place them on the line that represents time in your past.

2f: Now imagine joining your line of the future, present and past events.

3: Now remembering that negative attitude or a feeling you have. Imagine going backwards in time identifying times in your past where you had that negative feeling before. At each time you notice those negative feelings. Make a mental note and continue backwards to the very first experience you had of that attitude or feeling.

4: When you reach the very first experience of that attitude or feeling, detach yourself from the feeling and look at the memory from the left hand side.

See your younger self, what happened for you to feel these negative thoughts about yourself and the people around you.

Next step over the timeline to the right and look at the memory from another perspective.

Now imagine floating above the experience as high as you possibly can tell you can barely see it.

Now float back down and imagine going to a time shortly before the event which produced those feelings or attitude happened, you begin to realise those feelings were not always there. There was a time were you didn't have those negative feelings.

Gather all the information about what happened to make you feel this way from different perspectives, imagine walking or floating back alongside your timeline to the present.

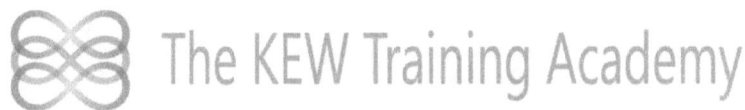
The KEW Training Academy

5: As you arrive at the present, look back along your Timeline of past events to that very first instance you experienced these negative feeling or attitudes. Determine what resources you have now at the age you are, life experience, and wisdom, you now have that would have been useful in that experience when you were younger. When you're young you do the best you can with the knowledge you have, though you are now older and you can deal with those feelings a lot better.

6: Fully associate into resources you have now i.e. confidence, intelligence, and wisdom, notice what you see, hear and feel when you're at your best. And Imagine filling up bag with all the positive resources you have now bringing them back to your past.

7: Now bring these resources back to your past. Imagine walking back alongside your Timeline in a place immediately before the memory of the past. Imagine passing all these resources back to the person you were when you first had these negative feelings about yourself, passing resources such as confidence, intelligence, experience, wisdom.

8: Having passed those resources to your younger self.

How is your response different to the experience you had that made you feel inadequate or negative?

How do you feel differently about yourself?

Now let those negative emotions go, let them go forever, your mind works to serve you and it may have been holding these thoughts to protect you though now it's time to let go.

Now picking up your balloon-exhale all those negative feelings into a balloon, get rid of those feelings into a balloon, blow it as big as you can, and imagine getting rid of every ounce of those negative feelings or attitude you had, once you have got rid of the negative feelings, tie the balloon up, and burst those feelings.

Now make your way back to the present having released all those negative feelings, and as you make your way back in time each time you come across the same negative feelings, release them, and replace them with the positive resources. As you make your way back to the present notice how you feel releasing all the negative energy.

9: Having released all the negative energy, imagine how you will respond differently to events and interactions with people. Having released your negative feelings, imagine 2 weeks into the future, then two months, 4 months, 6 months, then one year into the future laying down these new positive resources at each point.

10: Now from the future-face the present and notice the changes you have now made with those new positive resources, letting go of the old negative ones. Give your present self whatever information you have that will assist you in making those changes.

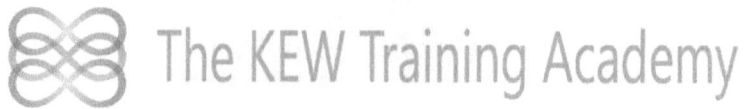

Now gradually come back into the here and now into the present feeling positive, refreshed recharged, focused and determined.

Train Journey - Time Line

Begin with your favourite induction and deepener.

Imagine your Time Line as a train journey - each station that you pass on the train represents a significant event or emotion in your life. The station that you're at now is the present time - on your journey through life.

Depending on where you want to reach - this could be a fast inter- city train or an older carriage that stops at every station - and the stations are actually named after the event or emotion that it symbolizes. For example, you may have a station called love or a station called first day at school - and the journey itself could be called your birth to the end of your life express - or it could go beyond to anything that happened in a previous life - or events of the future in an afterlife.

You're sitting next to the window on the train - and as you quickly pass a station you will see only fleeting glances of what happened at that one - but when your train stops you can see clearly and feel every emotion of that particular time in your life - but this time you will see it as an observer - and those emotions or events will have a totally different impact on you - for you are totally detached and relaxed.

Notice the direction that the train is taking - is it going from the past to the present or the present to the future or the present to the past? Is it going across country - from left to right? Or is it going up or down the country?

Be aware of your position on this train - you're in a comfortable seat - and the train is beginning to move - going to the first most significant event in your recent life - the problem that you've been experiencing - and as the train arrives at the station - you can see the name of the station or the emotion or wherever you are at this point in life.

What is the name of the station? (Wait for response) - Do you wish to stop and explore this memory?

(If yes - suggest that the memory begin to unfold - if no continue to another station)

(When an unpleasant or undesirable destination is reached, suggest that your client evaluate this situation rationally - if he or she cannot resolve it at this time, ask what they need and collect it from another station).

Continue by going through different stations - stopping where necessary - and collecting good feelings from past positive events and taking them to the ones that are causing difficulty in the client's life.

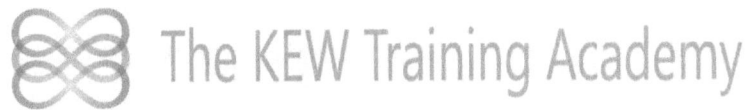

When the journey is finished - bring them back to the present station.

Pain & Healing Script

And now...as you become less aware of your physical body...you become more aware of your own perfect and pure subconscious mind....that really does know everything about you...and that subconscious part of you now opens....to receive...to accept and act on all the positive affirmations...concepts and images that I will suggest for you...as you drift deeper now.

As you drift deeper with every word that I speak...your subconscious mind is fully alert...active and alive both day and night...creating new energy....health and healing abilities allowing your body to rest...repair and regenerate...allowing you to adopt all those positive outlooks which are for your highest good and comfort.

Drifting even deeper now you allow your mind to become peaceful...calm and comfortable....as your body becomes rested...at ease...and now you can imagine yourself in a beautiful place...a place of comfort...peace and tranquillity...of safety and of healing...a warm woodland glade where you can feel comfortable...your mind and body rested...a place where you can return at any time...and you feel that you belong here...that you are valued and loved here...and those feeling comfort you so you are pleased to drift deeper now.

As you drift and move deeper into this place...the ground soft and springy beneath your step...the sunlight diffused by the branches and the foliage of the trees...the subtle sounds of the wonders of nature calming you....causing you to easily let go and rest so deeply now...you find yourself by a pool of crystal clear water...The pool is filled with natural spring water that is heated by nature's own forces....Steam rises from its gently bubbling surface...The pool looks so inviting and so comforting...restful and peaceful and you can begin to see...sense or imagine...yourself easing into the waters of the pool....you find a convenient rocky ledge that supports you and you feel so light...weightless here as the soothing waters rise to cover your chest and your shoulders....You have no concerns or fears....as the water bubbles around your body massaging and comforting every part of you.

The gentle heat of the waters relax you...soothe you...and you sense the gentle stimulation of the swirling waters....the bubbles massage your skin with a gentle penetrating warmth as the soft sensation surrounds you....penetrating deep into your muscles....into your bones...soothing your nerves....working on every cell and every fibre of your being....causing you to relax even more deeply than before as the waters swirl and the gentle heat penetrates deep within you...releasing all discomfort and pain...washed away by the gentle healing flow.

You relax even deeper now allowing the massaging effect of the healing waters to concentrate on those parts of you...joints and muscles that have been causing you pain and discomfort....and you feel those parts relax as the discomfort is soothed away....you experience a sense of release...freedom...peace and comfort that permeates your whole being.

You settle even deeper into relaxation now as the waters continue to massage....to calm and comfort you...every part of your body now is free of discomfort and of pain...you feel so comfortable now as pain and discomfort continue to flow away from you...your body becomes calmer....more peaceful...allowing itself to repair and heal...I am going to stop speaking now....allowing you some quiet time for yourself to continue to bathe in that soothing...warming water as it massages you and you continue now to allow all pain and discomfort to simply flow away.

(wait for a few minutes, allowing client to relax and enjoy the healing forces)

And now...you are feeling so rested...comforted...so completely relaxed....and you can see...sense or imagine yourself leaving the warm waters of the pool...knowing that you can return at any time...and as you lie down now on a grassy bank...the ground soft beneath you...supporting you...you feel warm and comfortable...tranquil and relaxed...gazing into the blue of the sky above...fixing your attention now onto a low cloud overhead.

The cloud acts for you like a cinema screen...and onto the screen you can see projected the image of your body...and you see this image with those areas of your body that have been causing you pain and discomfort...clearly defined...now your breathing slows...as your body rests...you see those areas clearly defined...now bathed in a warm and gentle...soft blue light...a light that surrounds those areas...covers those areas of discomfort...bathing them in a healing aura that begins to shrink...to diminish...and you know that as that healing aura begins diminishes...that light is absorbing all the causes and reasons for your discomfort...just as a sponge absorbs water....and you watch as these pools of light grow smaller and smaller...continuing to shrink with each outward breath...with each gentle beat of your heart....growing smaller now...as that sense of relief...of release...increases and you know that you are freeing yourself easily from discomfort now.

Allow the light to absorb more and more discomfort....drawing it in...cleansing freeing and leaving pleasurable sensations as the light shrinks down to just small dots...now you watch and observe the dots and the pain and discomfort contained within the dots...and as you watch...these dots burst open...changing to a gentle blue mist that flows outward from your body...rising towards the sun which evaporates them...eliminating them...and you feel totally free now.

And as you bring your attention back to the screen...you see that your body is completely bathed in white light now...the blue light is all gone and this white light acts as a silky...creamy ointment that lubricates your joints...soothes your muscles and cleanses every cell and every fibre of your being....your nerves are soothed and calmed...and every part of you continues to relax....and your perfect subconscious mind is instructed and activated now to make peace...relief and comfort...and freedom your natural way of being as it continues to work...night and day to make this reality...directing relief as and where needed....anticipating your body's needs...doing all that is needed to keep you comfortable and relaxed.

And now...as you continue to watch the screen...I want you to allow another image to appear...an image that represents the healing...comfort and release that has taken place...allow this image to develop....becoming clearer...more vivid...and now imagine this healing image becoming stronger now...more powerful...more vivid....Focus clearly and powerfully on this image and sense...Feel and imagine that it is taking place right in your body in just the right areas...let the sensation be one of healing...know that this is happening right now....and that healing...happiness and comfort continue within you whether you are here resting....sleeping or going about your daily activities...know that healing...comfort and pleasant sensations are your reality.

And so it is that healing...comfort...happiness and pleasant sensations **are** your reality...and you realise and understand that your body and mind are always alert...and if any situation arises within your body that requires your attention...then that information is communicated to you...quickly...accurately and with minimum of discomfort.

And your pure subconscious mind knows that once attention has been drawn to an area that needs attention...and that you have acknowledged that pain and discomfort are no longer productive...it will release them...allowing you to maintain your feelings of peace...relaxation and comfort.

I am now going to give you some trigger words...that will act as a post hypnotic conditioned response...whenever you want to boost your positive thinking...intensify your subconscious activity in producing good feelings...and wellness...you simply close your eyes...breathe deeply...exhale slowly and say to yourself...**easy control**....you breathe deeply...exhale slowly and you say to yourself...**easy control** and these words act as a conditioned response signal that informs your subconscious that it needs to create immediately...a feeling of wellness...feelings of freedom...comfort.

As you leave this place now...you feel yourself moving into a bright new day...a brand new day where you enjoy now...a feeling of lifted spirits...more positivity...an almost overwhelming sense of wellbeing...and you sense calm...acknowledge that you belong and that you are happy...that you can create your own reality now...and the following words...concepts...affirmations and images profoundly impress your pure and perfect subconscious mind...becoming activated now in your every thought and activity...natural behaviour.

- You are relaxed, calm and happy

- This is a good day for you...any discomfort is immediately released

- Your body relaxes naturally...each day as you practice your programmed relaxation...you become more relaxed...more skilled at relaxing and your deep signal

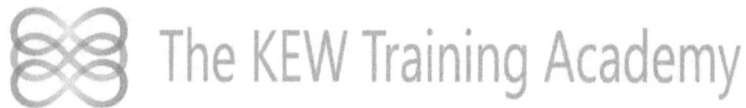
breath and your natural state of relaxation become effective protection against discomfort

- A new door in your life stands open before you now as you naturally see the best in all situations

- You deserve to be healthy...you deserve to be loved and you are a stronger, wiser person because of your experiences....because of the tests and challenges placed upon your mind and body

- Your thoughts are healing...nurturing...and you now release the past to make way for a glorious new present moment...love and healing fill and surround every cell and fibre of your being

- You are confident and optimistic as you say goodbye to the past fears and you embrace change...accepting that everything is part of your natural evolution...ultimately leading to your highest good

- You now release your fears and insecurities and replace them with faith and confidence

- You are free and you choose to accept peace...health and happiness...to be your natural condition

- Your sleep is relaxed and refreshed and you awake to each new day determined to live each moment in perfect happiness and joy

- You grow stronger and every day at a more subtle level...you are naturally healing

- Your cellular memory is focused now on positivity...on health and on wellbeing

- Your mind is charged with healing goals that permeate every cell of your body

- You feel good about yourself...day and night...directing healing thoughts and energies throughout your entire being...images...producing a satisfying...calmer and more productive life as you create joy...happiness and peace and calm in every waking moment....learning from the past...unafraid of the future...and happy in the only moment that has true meaning for you...the present one...a true gift to you.

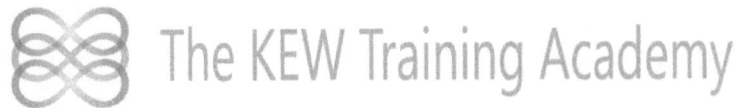

Glove Anaesthesia Hypnotherapy for Pain Management

The following hypnosis script can be used to assist a client with pain management. Use after induction & deepener.

Now that you are feeling more comfortable, I would like to show you how easily you can change sensations in your body by using your mind. In a moment I'll touch your hand. And as I touch your hand, you can let your focus on the sound of my voice, allow you to feel even more comfortable.

[begin touching lightly or tapping on the back of hand]

Just notice, as I touch your hand, that all sensations begin to change.. Many people notice a slight tingling sensation on that hand or elsewhere, maybe on your arm...or your face. Or somewhere else... But however you can experience this...all the things I do here on that hand.. .can allow you to feel even more comfort

You may be aware of my touch.. or not...and it might seem to be...over there. .kind of at a distance...

Imagine if you will, that this area...from the wrist to the fingertips is in a comfortable glove.....Very comfortable...custom made for you....and the area within begins to feel even more relaxed...more comfortable...You may think of this as your glove of relaxation....your glove of anaesthesia.....

And you might remember what that sensation feels like...the aspirin you might have had...in the past...And everywhere...in that glove....can feel different...and my touch can make you feel even more relaxed....all that I do here can cause you to feel more and more comfort...You may be aware of my touch...but all that I do allows you to go deeper and deeper into comfort and relaxation

[begin to pinch the hand, above or in the area of the web between thumb and forefinger. Begin slowly and increase the pressure as you continue to speak in soothing tones]

More and more comfortable....you may be aware of my touch .and you might be wondering what I am doing.....as you go deeper into this comfort,.. relaxing more and more.. Noticing the comfortable tingling....perhaps aware of the changing sensations as you relax deeper....

Allowing that comfort to spread... especially within your glove of comfort... Glove of anaesthesia of relaxation...[you can emerge from hypnosis or keep going to transfer feelings to the face and other parts of the body where relaxation is needed]

And you might want to allow that comfort to spread....to anywhere you need that comfort.....knowing that you can move that glove...to anywhere you want to feel

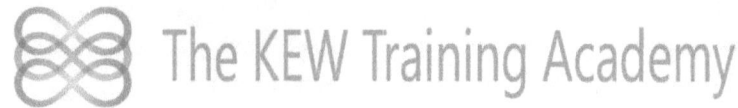

better...Notice what happens when I help you lift that glove to your face...how that sensation can spread...changing...that whole area can feel different more and more comfort spreading notice how easy you can bring that comfort to where you need it.. That's right....more and more comfortable , deeper and deeper relaxed .

[emerge slowly, allowing all sensations to return to normal or leaving comfort where patient needs it]

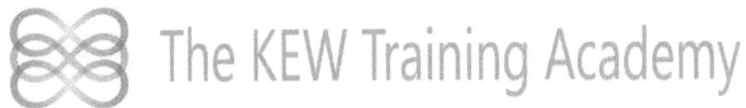

Hypnotic Writing for Business

How do you currently write your sales letters, emails, adverts and web site copy?

You already have a strategy for writing. So before we begin we need to understand how you currently go about your writing.

Explain your process.

What do you do just before you write?

What do you do as you write?

What do you do after you write?

Write your answers here:

....
....
....
....
....
....
....
....
....

Hypnotic Selling through Writing

Did mystery novelist Agatha Christie literally hypnotize her readers to buy her books?

According to a British television documentary aired in December 2005, scientists from three leading universities studied 80 of the famed novelists work and discovered she used words that invoked chemical responses in the brains of her readers.

The study called the Agatha Project involved loading Christies novels into a computer and analysing her words, phrases, and sentences. The scientists concluded that her phrases trigger a pleasure response. This causes people to seek out her books again and again, almost like an addiction.

According to the study Agatha used literary techniques mirroring those used by hypnotherapists and psychologists, which have a hypnotic effect on readers. The study found that common phrases used by Agatha act as a trigger to raise levels of serotonin and endorphins, the chemical messengers in the brain that induce pleasure.

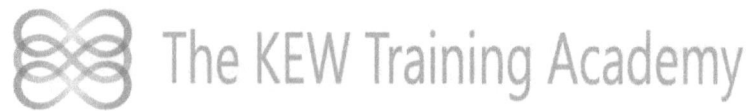
The KEW Training Academy

Certain words and phrases push buttons unconsciously in people, they respond without being aware of it, Using these following techniques you can improve your sales letters and website copy and the response that you get from readers.

People buy through EMOTION, all our behaviours are done through emotion.

When writing hypnotic copy you need to make sure that you translate your words in to something that is **meaningful, understandable and emotional.**

For example: You might turn the phrase:

"When was the last time you felt ok?" in to "When was the last time you felt fantastic?"

Every time you state a fact you need to describe to the reader just how this will benefit them. Get out of your ego and in to your readers ego, don't waffle on too much about yourself, always talk about the benefits your reader will get from having your product or service.

So what exactly is Hypnotic Writing?

Hypnotic Writing is a form of Waking Hypnosis.

"When hypnotic effects are achieved without the trance state, such hypnotic effects are called waking hypnosis." Dave Elman

Anything you do which makes your readers react because of MENTAL IMAGES you plant in their minds is HYPNOTIC WRITING.

Hypnotic writing is characterized by a focus of attention, It is a trance state where you are wide awake but focused on something you are reading.

Hypnotic writing achieves this state by the right use of words to create mental experiences. In other words, you get people so interested in your website, or e-mail, or sales letter that almost nothing else matters. And if you do this right, your **Hypnotic Writing will lead your readers to take action.**

Take a look at this pen below, it's a normal pen, it writes, and on the end of it it has a massaging head. You press it against your skin and you get a massage. It's not much to go on, but how would you write a paragraph to sell this pen?

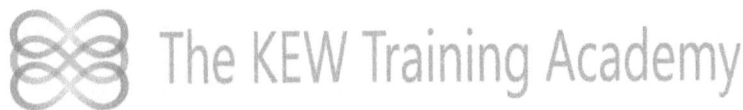

Here is how one website describes this pen:

Product Description: The unique metal ball-point pen with built-in massage. Rugged metal construction. Attractive design. Patented massage function. Replaceable ink refills Batteries included

Is that Hypnotic Writing?

No not at all.... Here is an example of Hypnotic Writing in action.

IMAGINE you had a teensy-weensy masseuse to carry around in your shirt pocket. Any time you desired, you could order your mini masseuse to soothe your tired muscles and rub away your tensions. Now imagine this tiny masseuse had a pen sticking out of his head and ran on batteries.

Well, you're not likely to come across a miniature, pen- headed masseuse – but here's the next best thing. Introducing the world's first MASSAGING PEN!!

OK, so why is this text Hypnotic?

....

....

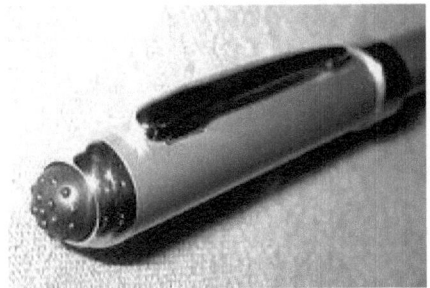

Hypnosis in Business & Selling

It has been said by many successful entrepreners throughout the ages that

"You can't go very far in business without learning a little hypnosis"

Understanding Hypnosis helps you to understand the mind of your reader. People are self-centered, that's not negative, that's reality. They walk around in their own trance, their bundle of experiences, beliefs, thoughts, and actions create a unique world where they live, move and breathe. Each of us, really is in our own hypnotic state.

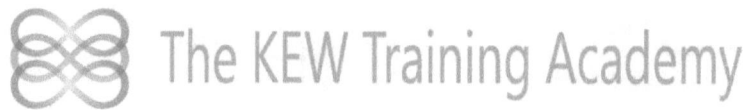

The first step in writing Hypnotic Copy is understanding the mind of your reader. That mind is not focused on your writing, that mind is absorbed with its own concerns. In order for you to make contact, you have to enter that mind where it already is.

In order to lead the reader in to a state of relaxed awareness – which is what hypnosis is – you have to meet them where they are mentally.

You have to meet the reader where their thoughts already are. You can do this with a headline that speaks to their problem or their dream. Then persuade people through your words moving them in to a buying trance.

Hypnotic ways to cause ACTION

When writing hypnotic copy for your website, sales letters, emails etc there is a formula to follow.

Formula for Persuasion:

1. **Problem**

2. **Promise**

3. **Proof**

4. **Price**

Start off by asking yourself these questions:

1. Are you getting attention with your opening?

2. Are you stating a problem the reader cares about? 3. Are you offering a solution that really works?

3. Are you asking the reader to take action?

PROBLEM

Begin your writing with a headline that calls out the audience you want by focusing on their problem. For example, if you are selling a weight loss product of some sort, you might use a headline such as:

Want to lose weight?

What you are doing is rounding up the people who will want to buy from you by focussing on their problem or issue.

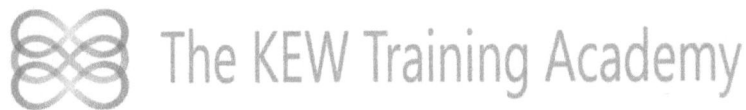

If you are a massage therapist with your own site, your headline at the top of your website might read:

Stressed/ Want to release your tension in 30 minutes or less?

Ask yourself, what is the problem my visitors are having? Whatever it is, you then create a main headline at the top of your website or sales letters etc that speaks to it.

PROMISE

You've got your readers attention with step one, now you need to mention your promise.

e.g/ New non diet approach relies on your mind, not your food, to lose weight fast.

And the massage therapist example might read;

My hands have eased 3,500 bodies just like yours, I can help you too...

In this second step you are explaining HOW you can solve the problem stated in step one. If you are truly focused on their problem, you will be putting them into a waking trance with Hypnotic Writing.

PROOF

Next you need proof as we live in an age of scepticism. These can be in the form of testimonials, a guarantee or anything else that you can think of that will convince people you are being honest with them.

An example might be:

Research shows people lose on average 4lbs per week with this new plan.

You will feel so relaxed from my massage that you will fall asleep on my table.

Here you need to bring in your evidence that your promise will work.

PRICE

Finally you need to ask for what you want. If you want people to sign up for your newsletter, say so. If you want them to buy your product, say so. If you want them to call you, say so. People want to be led, but they won't take action unless you spell it out for them, and tell them the price for doing so.

Eg. If you don't take care of that back pain, what might the results be long term? Call us Today to book your Free Consultation.

Exercise:

Hypnotherapy Practitioner Course - Professional Accredited Hypnotherapy Training

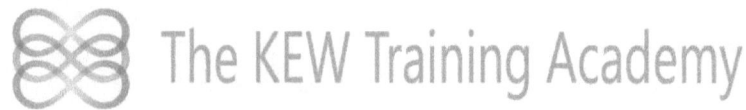

Think about your own service or product that you are looking to sell and have a practice writing Hypnotic Copy.

Notes:

What Every Reader Wants to Know

If you give people what they want they will listen to you. What does every reader want in your writing? People generally ask themselves a few questions when they pick up something to read. Here they are;

"Who   cares?"
"So   what?"
"What's in it for me?"

You need to know the answers to these questions. What is in it for the reader? What are his benefits? What will he get out of it? Why should he care about what you've written?

"Who cares?" (Well who does care about your writing? Why should they care?) "So what?" (Well, so what? Why does your writing matter? Do you have something important to say? It is *really* important?)

"What's in it for me?" (Well, what is in it for him? What will he get out of your writing?)

You have to put your feet in to the other person's shoes. Imagine what they want. Rapport is a key to any success in selling.

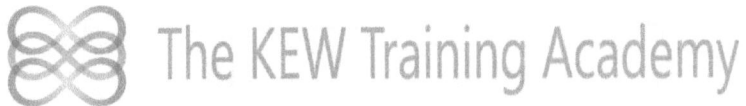
The KEW Training Academy

Group Sessions

Deciding to do Group Hypnotherapy sessions can be a great idea. You can do group sessions for issues like Stop Smoking, Losing Weight and Stress Management.

In this scenario, you would have a group of people that all had the same issue that they would want solving, example of Stop Smoking. You would then get the group together and Hypnotise them all at the same time. You could find out the common goals of what they wanted to achieve, do the Induction and put in the suggestions that they stop smoking, live a healthy life etc.

Group sessions can be a great way of more people coming along to see you, they may want to have 1-2-1 sessions with you afterwards and in the group session, as you have more people, you charge less and it works out to be more cost effective for the client's.

Essential Marketing Tips for Getting Started with Clients

Know Your Customers' Needs . Things you need to know about your customers

- **Why they buy:** If you know why customers buy a product or service, it's easier to match their needs to the benefits your business can offer.

- **When they buy:** If you approach a customer just at the time they want to buy, you will massively increase your chances of success.

- **How they buy:** For example, some people prefer to buy from a website, while others prefer a face-to-face meeting.

- **How much money they have:** You'll be more successful if you can match what you're offering to what you know your customer can afford.

- **What makes them feel good about buying:** If you know what makes them tick, you can serve them in the way they prefer.

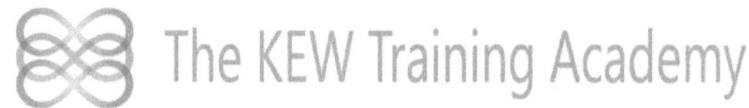

- **What they expect of you:** For example, if your customers expect reliable delivery and you don't disappoint them, you stand to gain repeat business.

- **What they think about your competitors:** If you know how your customers view your competition, you stand a much better chance of staying ahead of your rivals. Generate business from your e-marketing plan, promoting your website, direct navigation

- **What they think about you:** If your customers enjoy dealing with you, they're likely to buy more. And you can only tackle problems that customers have if you know what they are.

There are three main ways that people arrive at websites – direct navigation, web referrals and search engines.

Web referrals: Web referrals are an important means of attracting visitors to your site. There are a number of ways you can generate these.

- Include your web address in all email footers.

- Email marketing - targeted electronic newsletters and offers to customers can be very effective. If the offer is interesting it is easy for people to pass the email on.

- Online advertising - the use of banner and pop-up adverts on other websites to drive people to yours

- Reciprocal marketing - finding sites with complementary content and agreeing to have links or banners to each other's sites.

- Forums - you can set up your own, or monitor others, join the discussion and point people towards your website

Search engines

While search engines are far outstripped by direct referrals, they can still prove useful for attracting customers. Competition for a high ranking on the major search engines is intense because few web users look beyond the second page of results.

If you are expecting your website to generate significant commercial returns, it will be well worth spending the time and effort to ensure you get the most out of your search engine placement.

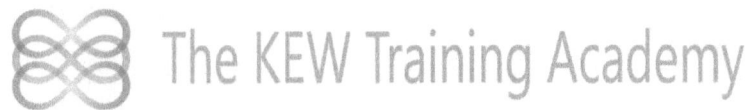

Generate business from your e-marketing plan & Email marketing

More and more people have an email address that allows them to receive documents or other files electronically. It is a fast, flexible and effective way of getting marketing messages through - such as newsletters or special offers - without the time lag and costs associated with printing.

It's essential not to overuse email marketing. What makes it so effective - the personal, time-sensitive interaction - can also irritate people if it is irrelevant or unwanted.

You should also consider compatibility. Different programs will display email differently. An email with images or an HTML component could look messy on a different set-up, or even cause the program to crash.

The solution is to profile your customers and understand what the best format is for them. Some may like high-tech e-marketing, others might prefer a plain-text email.

Email marketing rules

In December 2003, new rules came into force covering marketing emails to individuals. The Privacy and Electronic Communications Regulations introduced an **opt-in** consent procedure for commercial emails - which means you can only target people who have agreed to be contacted.

Advantages of email marketing

- Flexible - you can send plain text, graphics or attach files -whichever suits your message best.

- Easy for people to forward on to others, building your reputation by word of mouth.

- People can click on links and follow your call to action immediately.

- Less intrusive than telephone marketing.

- Files need to be small enough to download quickly.

- Unsolicited commercial email or "spam" irritates consumers. You need to make sure that your email marketing complies with privacy and data protection rules, and that it is properly targeted at people who want to receive it.

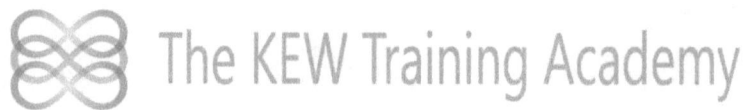

Advertising and sponsorship

Banner adverts

Pay search engines to include your website as a **sponsored link**. Sponsored links appear at the top or on the right-hand side of the search results. To become a sponsored link you bid for particular keywords or phrases. Your ranking is determined by how much you pay each time your link is clicked - known as "cost-per-click" pricing. You can set your own daily budget to help you control costs and once your daily budget is spent your ad is turned off until the next day. You may have to pay an initial set-up cost and set up an account to cover the costs incurred.

Use the web tools provided by the search engines to help you improve your website's ranking. Many of the main search engines - such as Google, Ask, Yahoo and MSN - provide tips, advice and tools to help you improve your website's usability.

Banners and buttons occupy designated space for rent on web pages. They are similar to the print advertising model used by newspapers and magazines, except they can include video, audio and interactive capabilities in just a few square inches of space.

Most banners work on the basis of click-trough's, the user clicks on the banner and is linked through to the website that is paying for the advert.

Banners can be useful for brand awareness, but response rates tend to be very low.

Sponsorship

Many businesses are developing partnerships with website owners to combine useful content with advertising. This content may contain references to their own products or services. Alternatively the web page itself can include advertising links through to their own website.

The sponsorship approach can work particularly well where the quality of the editorial content is high, or where the website is recognised as a good independent source of information. As with traditional magazines, the advertorial approach of blatantly plugging your own business can quickly put readers off.

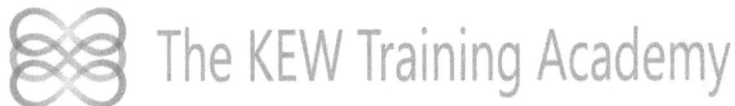
The KEW Training Academy

Essential Websites for Marketing your Business and Getting a Presence on the Internet

Email Marketing, Building Database Lists www.getresponse.com or www.constantcontact.com
Free 30 day trial

Wordpress – Free Websites and Blogs www.wordpress.com

Facebook – Add the link of your company facebook profile to your website www.facebook.com

Twitter – Update your free twitter account daily to attract customers and keep existing clients informed and updated about what's happening with your business www.twitter.com

Linked In – Fill in your company details, what you do and what services you offer www.linkedin.com

Free business cards, leaflets etc www.vistaprint.com

Directories

www.thomsondirectories.com www.freeindex.co.uk

Useful Information

⬜ British Institute of Hypnotherapy (BIH) Tel: 01702 524 484

Website:http://www.britishinstituteofhypnotherapy-nlp.com/

Balens Insurance: http://www.balens.co.uk/

Phone **01684 580 776**

Email mailto:commercial@balens.co.uk

Hypnotherapy Scripts www.hypnoticworld.com

Other useful websites:

Royalty Free Music - http://www.silenciomusic.co.uk/ Facebook www.facebook.com

Hypnotherapy Practitioner Course - Professional Accredited Hypnotherapy Training

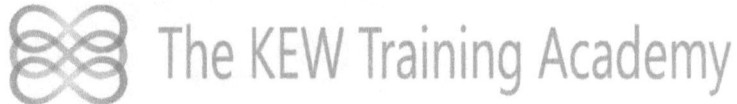

Recommended Reading List

- **Training Trances -** by John Overdurf and Julie Silverthorn

- **Scripts and Strategies in Hypnotherapy: The Complete Works**
  -by Roger P. Allen

- **The Intention Experiment** by Lynn McTaggart

- **Hypnotherapy for Dummies** by Mike Bryant and Peter Mabbutt

- **Hypnotherapy Scripts: A Neo-Ericksonian Approach to Persuasive Healing** by Ronald A. Havens and Catherine Walters

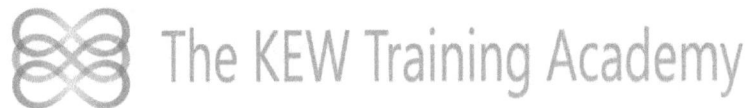
The KEW Training Academy

Hypnotherapy Practitioner Programme

Assessment Questions

Marks that are available for each question appear in brackets

1. Describe in your own words what you understand hypnosis to be. (5)

2. Explain the different parts of the mind and their main functions. (10)

3. Which part of the mind is in control and why? (2)

4. Discuss the different kinds of brain wave activity and when we tend to go in to those states. (10)

5. Give a brief history of the development of hypnosis over the years. (10)

6. What is calibration and why is it so important to use it with clients. (10)

7. Explain the different types of hypnosis and include what kind of client would respond best to each type. (8)

8. Outline the key points to structuring a successful appointment? (4)

9. Read through the sample weight loss questionnaire. If this was your client, what key things would you be looking for in their answers in the questionnaire? (4)

10. Often when a client comes to see you for a specific problem such as weight loss there can be many other things going on at a deeper level. Re-read through the sample weight loss questionnaire and see what other issues appear to be apparent in the responses given. (8)

11. What is a pre-talk/consultation and why do we use one? (3)

12. List the ways in which we can build rapport with clients. (6)

13. Why do we use suggestibility tests? (2)

14. Practice both suggestibility tests on at least 2 people and note your findings. (4)

15. Discuss the various styles of hypnotic inductions and give a short example of how each may be used. (8)

16. What must all inductions bring about? (5)

17. Discuss the different types of language used in inductions. (8)

Hypnotherapy Practitioner Course - Professional Accredited Hypnotherapy Training

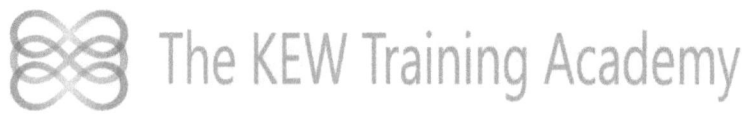

18. List the structure to an induction. (8)

19. Re-write 3 of any of the sample induction scripts using some of the hypnotic language off the hypnotic language sheets, put them in your own words for use with future clients.(24)

20. Re-write 2 of any of the deepener scripts using hypnotic language and put them in to your own style of speaking that will help you deliver them with ease. (24)

21. Practice each induction and deepener script that you have re- written, with a willing subject and note your findings. Concentrate on practicing your voice tone and tempo, rhythm and collaboration.(30)

22. Practice a full weight loss session with a client. Note which techniques you used and the feedback from the client. What did you learn throughout the session? What would you do differently next time? (if anything) (30)

23. Practice a full smoking cessation session with a client, note which techniques you used and the feedback from the client. What did you learn throughout the session? What would you do differently next time? (if anything) (30)

24. Practice a full phobia cure session with a client, note which techniques you used and the feedback from the client. What did you learn throughout the session? What would you do differently next time? (if anything) (30)

25. Practice a full stress relief session with a client, note which techniques you used and the feedback from the client. What did you learn throughout the session? What would you do differently next time? (if anything) (30)

Please complete the assessment questions and return to:

The KEW Training Academy, 8 Stockley Mews, Shevington, Wigan WN6 8AN

Please remember to enclose your name & address for certification.